Overall, this read is excellent as paradigmatic of the analyst's task to continually revisit the old with new eyes and, as White points out, to be mindful of the multiplicity of conceptual and perceptual frameworks that any approach to the psyche must embrace. White's foray into his topic exemplifies how a sharp and open mind can simultaneously observe and participate in an important theme and highlight a world lying hidden within it. What is most impressive is that even with such hovering clarity, White always draws us back to earth, back to what is before us. His sparkling insights, grounded in philosophical understanding, become not only accessible, but immediately useful."

—Mark Dean, MA, ATR-BC, LPC, president,
Philadelphia Association of Jungian Analysts

"A gem of a book that, in its originality, scholarship, practicality, and thorough analysis, unfailingly enriches one's theoretical and clinical perspectives—including, and not least poignantly, on oneself."

—Randall Hoedeman, PhD, LPC, LMFT,
AAMFT-approved supervisor

New Imago: Series in Theoretical, Clinical, and Applied Psychoanalysis

Series Editor

Jon Mills, Adler Graduate Professional School, Toronto

New Imago: Series in Theoretical, Clinical, and Applied Psychoanalysis is a scholarly and professional publishing imprint devoted to all aspects of psychoanalytic inquiry and research in theoretical, clinical, philosophical, and applied psychoanalysis. It is inclusive in focus, hence fostering a spirit of plurality, respect, and tolerance across the psychoanalytic domain. The series aspires to promote open and thoughtful dialogue across disciplinary and interdisciplinary fields in mental health, the humanities, and the social and behavioral sciences. It furthermore wishes to advance psychoanalytic thought and extend its applications to serve greater society, diverse cultures, and the public at large. The editorial board is comprised of the most noted and celebrated analysts, scholars, and academics in the English-speaking world and is representative of every major school in the history of psychoanalytic thought.

Titles in the Series

Praise for *Adaptation and Psychotherapy: Langs and Analytical Psychology*

"Owing to recent the decline of ego-psychology, adaptation has become a neglected topic in the analytic literature. John White gives the term (in its various significations) renewed relevance to clinical work through a remarkable synthesis of ideas gleaned from Carl Jung and Robert Langs. White delves deep into their core similarities and differences, their strengths, weaknesses, and blind spots, demonstrating how they complement each other in striking ways. What makes Dr. White's effort so memorable, original, and persuasive is the deep historical and philosophical knowledge that he brings to bear on these reflections—a trait which is usually absent in the clinical literature—and his ability to salvage and build upon the now all-but-forgotten legacy of a brave, brilliant, but idiosyncratic man like Robert Langs. Here's hoping this book will give Langs's work a renewed lease on life."

—Daniel Burston, Duquesne University,
author of *The Wing of Madness,*
The Life and Work of R. D. Laing and *The Legacy of Erich Fromm*

"John White writes as I imagine he teaches—patiently circling back at orchestrated intervals to summarize the rich ground he has tilled in his scrupulously linear and scholarly text. In introducing Jungians to Langs and bridging the contributions of Jung and Langs to the theory of adaptation, White breathes new life into and highlights the relevance of adaptation to clinical practice for Jungians and psychoanalysts alike, supplementing Jung's Psychology with Langsian innovations (e.g., in his discussion of Langs's seminal notion of "derivatives") while reiterating the timeless resonance of Jung's broader and ultimately deeper conception of individuation, as the movement of the Self, in the lifelong adaptive process of psychic development. White's achievement here in 'bringing these two approaches into something like harmony, without overlooking their incompatibilities,' is nuanced and deft, like that of the experienced teacher who somehow gleans new harvest from well-trodden earth."

—Laura C. Tuley, LPC, PhD, coordinator,
The New Orleans Jungian Seminar

"Guided by Robert Langs and Carl Jung as they complement, deepen, and correct each other's work, John White clearly and comprehensively explores that vital dynamic at the heart of life and, thus, of effective psychotherapy: the nature and process of authentic adaptation. Further guided by his training as both a philosopher and an analyst, he convincingly does so at the borders of psychoanalytic theory, metapsychology, philosophy, clinical 'technique,' and the lifelong challenge of being and becoming more wholly human. In the process, he better introduces Jung to the Freudian community, and Langs, including the totality of his work, to the Jungian community (as well as each to his own

community!). Clinical illustrations include a highly engaging case study of derivative listening around the adaptive context of a tape recorder. The result is a gem of a book that, in its originality, scholarship, practicality, and thorough analysis, unfailingly enriches one's theoretical and clinical perspectives—including, and not least poignantly, on oneself."
—Randall Hoedeman, PhD, LPC, LMFT,
AAMFT-approved supervisor

"White's work in *Adaptation and Psychotherapy* is an important contribution to psychoanalysis, analytical psychology, and compara- tive psychoanalysis. No other author has offered a comparison of the theoretical systems of both C. G. Jung and Robert Langs in the history of psychoanalysis. White brings the ongoing relevance of these two significant figures into sharp focus, particularly their relevance to contemporary practice. Offering a unique perspective on the theories of both men, White outlines the central importance of the patient's capac- ity for adaptation in analytic treatment and how the treatment process is deepened by a focus on adaptation. In doing so, he provides a fresh look at the theories of both men and the ways the two systems are complementary. Psychoanalysis as a field benefits from the kind of rigorous, careful analysis of core concepts that John White provides in this volume."
—Mark Winborn, licensed clinical psychologist and
nationally certified psychoanalyst

"A thought-provoking and well-presented development of a synthesis of the contrasting approaches to adaptation found in the works of Robert J. Langs and Carl G. Jung. This work provides an important bridge between conflicting theories of the human psyche and the different therapeutic approaches based upon these theories. The philosophical, theoretical, and clinical perspec- tives are considered as central concerns of psychotherapeutic healing. This book has the potential to advance the science and art of analytic training and supervision for analysts of all analytic persuasions."
—Douglas R. Cann, PhD, CPsych,
Jungian analyst, private practice

"White has utilized a scrutiny of Robert Langs's understanding of adaptation as a springboard to bring clarity to some key issues facing the psychotherapists of our era. White illuminates a diversified perspective, freeing adaptation from a one-sided historical or causal understanding, or one of simple acquiescence to context, and linking it to possibilities inherent in the individual and in nature. At its heart, this is a work about clarity which, to White's credit, draws us into a more pluralistic grasp of psychological phenomena—a notion that points back to the necessity of the continual growth of the theorist or therapist demanded by psychological work.

ADAPTATION AND PSYCHOTHERAPY

Langs and Analytical Psychology

John R. White

ROWMAN & LITTLEFIELD
Lanham • Boulder • New York • London

Published by Rowman & Littlefield
An imprint of The Rowman & Littlefield Publishing Group, Inc.
4501 Forbes Boulevard, Suite 200, Lanham, Maryland 20706
www.rowman.com

86-90 Paul Street, London EC2A 4NE

British Library Cataloguing in Publication Information Available

Library of Congress Cataloging-in-Publication Data

Names: White, John R., 1953- author.
Title: Adaptation and psychotherapy : Langs and analytical psychology / John R. White, PhD, LPC, Duquesne University.
Description: Lanham : Rowman & Littlefield, [2023] | Series: New imago: series in theoretical, clinical, and applied psychoanalysis | Includes bibliographical references and index.
Identifiers: LCCN 2022042240 (print) | LCCN 2022042241 (ebook) | ISBN 9781538117934 (cloth) | ISBN 9781538117941 (paperback) | ISBN 9781538117958 (epub)
Subjects: LCSH: Langs, Robert, 1928-2014. | Psychotherapy. | Adaptability (Psychology) | Jungian psychology.
Classification: LCC RC480 .W485 2023 (print) | LCC RC480 (ebook) | DDC 616.89/14--dc23/eng/20221114

LC record available at https://lccn.loc.gov/2022042240

LC ebook record available at https://lccn.loc.gov/2022042241

To my wife, Kristy,
and to the memory of Robert J. Langs

Brief Contents

Contents

Acknowledgments

A work of this kind owes much to many people—colleagues, friends, patients, family members, and others—not all of whom, unfortunately, can be acknowledged by name in this space.

My first thanks go to my former counseling supervisor and my current friend and colleague, Randall Hoedeman. It was a strange coincidence—or was it a felicitous synchronicity?—which resulted in my using Randy's office on Thursdays during my final semester of internship, while still supervising with him. One fateful Wednesday at noontime, during our supervision hour, I asked Randy about the author of some fifteen books I had noticed on his shelf, "Robert Langs, I think, is his name." "Oh . . . Langs? . . . you've never heard of Langs? Well . . . he has a lot to say about what we were just talking about." We had just been talking about a patient of mine, and Randy had been highlighting issues associated with what I now know of as the therapeutic frame and communicative fields. Randy then pointed to a series of Langs' supervision transcripts and suggested I begin with one (which I did), *The Listening Process*, while I was using his office on Thursdays, in between patients. That was the original experience of Langs which soon engendered the idea of writing a book on adaptation in Langs and Jung. I am still deeply grateful for the many hours—both within supervision and without—that Randy and I talked about Langs and his relevance to clinical practice, not to mention the hundreds of emails we exchanged with some reference to Langs. This book would not have happened had it not been for those events and for those many happy hours of discussion—not to mention outstanding supervision—with Randy.

I owe a similar debt of gratitude to my former analytic supervisor, Sandra Miller, and to my former analyst, Stanton Marlan. As has always been the case for his readers, studying Langs challenged me a good deal, especially since I was first reading his work intensely while going through the formative time and process of Jungian analytic training. Sandy's consistent willingness to allow me to work through Langs' teaching and consistent invitation to compare and contrast Langs' and Jung's (and White's!) approach set much of the background and tone of this work. Stan, for his part, guided me through the self-doubts, the emotional disturbances, and the identity crises Langs' teaching brought with it, of which there were more than a few.

Thanks are due to three outstanding analysts who read earlier versions of this work: Mark Winborn, Marilyn Matthews, and August Cwik. Their consistent support, encouragement, interest, and excellent critical comments were deeply appreciated. Thanks also to the various analysts and analysts-in-training with whom I had discussions about Langs early on, especially Paul Kugler, Mark Dean, Ron Curran, Michelle Cooper, and Larry Rayburn. These five may not even recall those discussions, but they should know that they contributed in significant ways to early formulations of a number of ideas still extant in this book. I am also extremely grateful to the facilitating analysts—Constance Romero, Tim Pilgrim, and Charles Zeltzer—as well as to my excellent peers, through my years of control colloquium, both for their responses to my thoughts and for their patience as I worked through some of my ideas on Langs with reference to our cases. Thanks also to Thomas Janoski, formerly president of the Pittsburgh Psychoanalytic Center, for his invitation to present a part of this work at the Pittsburgh Psychoanalytic Center in April 2018, and to the many people who attended and commented. This Jungian always feels very welcomed by the excellent Freudian analysts and candidates who are associated with the center. Thanks also to my colleagues at the Pittsburgh Pastoral Institute, to whom I presented parts of this work in March of 2017.

Special thanks go to my former patient, whom I call "Bruce," who was more than willing to permit me to discuss some of his personal material from our sessions for the purposes of illustration. Thanks also go to the many unnamed patients who do not know how much they have aided me in my understanding of adaptation and its clinical relevance.

I also want to thank both Daniel Burston and Sharna Olfman who, through some very challenging years, were among my chief supports, in too many ways to list here. Also, a sincere word of thanks goes to James Swindal and to Jeff McCurry of Duquesne University, who invited me to be a "Scholar-in-Residence" at the university for a number of semesters, allowing me among other things full access to the Duquesne's excellent library and wonderful library staff.

Thanks also to my two stepchildren, Meghan and Branden, who gave me the opportunity to be a stepfather and from whom I learned so very much about adaptation, as I had the privilege of watching them develop from children into wonderful adults.

Finally, I need to thank the two people who, more than any others, made this work possible and to whom the book is dedicated. The first is the late Robert Langs, with whom I was in email correspondence during the early years of the formulation of this book and the last three-plus years of his life, until his death on November 8, 2014. A few months after my first experience of reading Langs' work, in June 2011, I found an email address for Langs at the bottom of one of his articles and took the risk of writing him an email that was half "question from a student" and half fan mail. His response appeared twenty-five minutes later, and our mutual correspondence continued from that point on. We stayed in fairly consistent communication, usually corresponding at least once a week, even if it was no more than asking how the other was doing, until Bob's death. While Bob and I usually talked about his theory and only talked very indirectly about patients, the ongoing interaction with him and his availability when I had questions or doubts about his thinking was of course a great help to my understanding of his work and to the application of his thought in my own clinical practice. Also, Bob's humble request that I create a Wikipedia article for him gave me an opportunity to take a broad look at his work, while also giving me a concrete way of thanking him for his availability. When I would speak a bit of some of my thoughts on his work that have since entered into this book, he was as a rule unhappy with them. Yet he was always simultaneously supportive and interested, and always gracious even as he expressed his doubts. I'm not sure how to put into words all that that correspondence meant to me, but I can say that having the experience of corresponding with Bob while studying his work enacted many and profound changes in me, as a person and as an analyst-in-training. Though I certainly experienced some of the brusqueness, mild aggression, and feelings of not being appreciated for which Bob was famous, I saw other things in him as well that I've not seen noted elsewhere, such as his excellent sense of humor and his worldly wisdom. He was unassuming enough to handle my teasing him (like when I suggested I should put a picture of Cary Grant rather than his own on his Wikipedia page) and was typically warm, lighthearted, affirming, and willing to share what insights he had about analysis and in fact about life from his own experience—traits rarely mentioned about him but which in my experience were at least as important as the others. I am deeply grateful that I had those opportunities.

The other person who made this book possible is my wife, Kristy, who accompanied me throughout the entire process of the writing of this book. Indeed, she helped me not only as my emotional support and partner but also by being an outstanding librarian. Kristy, more than anyone else, knows how much of myself I invested in all aspects of this book, in all its iterations, and how many challenges there were—whether associated with my first interactions with Langs, or with my early efforts to internalize his ideas, or with trying to write while going through training, obtaining counseling licensure, and changing professions from philosophy professor to psychoanalyst, or with the emotional disturbances around my own analytic identity . . . and so many others. Kristy alone knows all about these because she generously shared them with me, often reminding me, in her inimitable way, who I really am and what I was really about, and encouraging me to continue down my own path.

Preface

In the early 1970s, someone who would turn out to be a major figure in American psychoanalysis suddenly burst upon the analytic scene. His name was everywhere it seemed—as the author of books and articles, in book reviews in Freudian and Jungian journals, in announcements of presentations and supervision seminars he was to give at prestigious training institutions, in the position of editor of journals and book series. His name was also to be found in innumerable articles and article titles, authored both by people who admired him and by those who sought to "bring him down a peg or two." There were, in fact, quite a few of the latter. For he was not a man to be trifled with: he had enormous intellectual energy coupled with a large dose of ambition; in his seminars, he could be warm and humorous yet also demanding and at times devastatingly critical; he was impassioned, narcissistic (by his own admission), at times aggressive; he had a great deal of confidence in what he saw and yet displayed that same confidence, even if his opinion was quite the opposite of what he had adamantly asserted a short time previously.

He fought hard to preserve the genuine spirit of the psychoanalytic tradition that he loved so passionately, yet he also sought to alter that tradition by underlining an element of psychoanalytic clinical theory that he thought was underrated. He wrote literally thousands of pages, taught, and gave lectures to the tune of hundreds of hours, ironically enough so he could teach analysts and therapists how to listen. And having fulfilled a dream and risen to the heights of the psychoanalytic world in the 1970s and 1980s, his dream was more or less completely shattered by the late 1990s and never returned. He died on November 8, 2014, feeling mostly a forgotten man. He was nothing if not a man of paradox and contradictions, contradictions which in many ways defined his professional career and the passions which drove it.

I never met Robert J. Langs—the man I just described—in person, though I did correspond with him by email for over three years, right up to the time of his death. In fact, I didn't know for certain that he had died until three months after his death, when I noticed someone had added his death date to the Wikipedia article I had created for Langs some years previous. Though our email correspondence occurred near the end of his life, Langs was still to the end all the things I described here, often all of them together, even if in the diluted form that often comes with advanced age. By the time I corresponded with him, Langs felt himself a totally forgotten man, blacklisted and ignored, and he was eager for a new and open ear like mine.

Langs' perception of his place in the psychoanalytic world after the 1990s was in large measure correct: he was in many ways forgotten, except as a cautionary tale, with stories of his fall from grace and hypotheses concerning why he lost nearly all his patients at one point. Yet perhaps now, a few years after his passing and from a point in the history of depth psychology very different from the one that initiated his own trajectory, we can begin not only to look at the work of Robert Langs again, but also begin to evaluate and assimilate it. That Langs was such a public and controversial figure for some fifteen or twenty years probably impacted the extent to which his work was genuinely understood, as well as the extent to which it was both fairly and critically evaluated. I hope this study to be a step toward initiating the broader rethinking and reevaluating Langs' massive corpus of writings that I believe it deserves.

Why do I think Langs deserves such a reexamination? There are, I believe, a number of good reasons for revisiting Langs' work, among which I would highlight the following. First, I believe that Langs' intended corrective of psychoanalysis, one which underlined *adaptation* as a key to understanding psychic conflict and unconscious communication, really needed to be made. One is perhaps less likely to recognize the value of Langs' point in our own time if, for no other reason, because of the advent and dominance of relational psychoanalysis—an approach which in some ways arises in the wake of Langs' interactional approach to psychoanalytic psychotherapy, but in other ways flies in the face of it (e.g., by tending to reduce the significance of personal unconscious communication in favor of what is discovered in the therapeutic relationship). Yet the different emphases of contemporary psychoanalysis should not blind us to the ways in which a more classical form of analysis might not be entirely *passé* and, especially after years of being in some level of abeyance, might in our own time be once again a source of original thought.

A further reason is that, in my view, Langs' approach to psychoanalytic practice revealed a good deal more about depth psychology than Langs himself thought. Despite Langs' insistence on the importance of his approach, there are actually potentials in it that Langs himself did not see. This last point, I suggest, was in part due to the relatively impoverished understanding of the psyche that Langs had for at least most of his career, something I will return to frequently in the main body of this text. Briefly, it seems to me that Langs' understanding of his own "adaptive paradigm" was relatively and unnecessarily narrow, a classic case of a groundbreaking thinker and practitioner who did not fully appreciate the value of his own central insight.

Third, as alluded to previously, there is an important emphasis in Langs' work that has tended to become dulled in both Freudian and Jungian conceptions of psychoanalysis in our time, namely, the focus on unconscious communication. Though it might be plausible to say that Langs overemphasized unconscious communication, at least to the extent that he tended to think unconscious communication to be something like the sole principle guiding psychoanalytic work, there are grounds for thinking there is not enough emphasis on unconscious communication in our own time, especially of the more "everyday" variety found in derivative communication, in favor of more "conscious level" approaches to the psyche. It seems to me that, in our own time, Langs' emphasis is once again pertinent to analytic practice and in need of some new, careful, and critical consideration.

With these points in mind, the following text is intended to highlight certain core features of Langs' work, evaluate those features, and then treat what is best in Langs' theory in a broader, more expansive light. It is also intended to show, on the one hand, that the method Langs articulated for working clinically is basically correct but that, on the other, it is only a part of a broader clinical whole, something he did not clearly see.

My attempt to expand Langs' thought will also entail realigning his thought with the thought of another outstanding thinker and practitioner in the analytic tradition, namely, Carl Jung. Langs himself was cognizant of Jung's work and, as his career moved to its latter half, he studied Jung in more detail. For example, in his final published book, *Freud on a Precipice*, Langs makes use of Jung's archetypal theory as a way of explaining his own central theses concerning trauma and death anxiety. Nonetheless, Langs did not, so far as I know, link his clinical theory to Jung's conception of the structural statements of the psyche. Yet it is particularly in connection to Jung's richer conception of the psyche that Langs' clinical theory shows its real breadth. Hence, I will be linking Langs' clinical theory with Jung's conception of the psyche, something Langs himself did not do.

As a consequence of bringing Langs and Jung together, I will try to show not only that Langs was correct in thinking that adaptation is a central factor in psychic conflict—and thus equally central for analytic practice—but that we need both a more expansive notion of adaptation than Langs worked with and a deeper understanding of the psyche and psychic processes than Langs originally countenanced. Yet in that process, we will not lose the essence of Langs' teaching but find that his insights concerning adaptation, as well as the concomitant features of his paradigm, such as the importance of the analytic frame, reading derivative communications, and unconscious validation, are just as useful as he claimed they were.

This book is the first of its kind, in a number of respects. It is, first of all, the only book-length study to date which includes a substantial distillation of Robert Langs' adaptive clinical theory as a whole, in the form of a single, coherent text (chapter 3) and viewed from the standpoint of his entire corpus of writings.[1] This was not a simple endeavor, because Langs' work is often serpentine and "in process." Thus, two in some ways contrasting difficulties arise in trying to understand Langs' thought: (1) on the one hand, Langs' thought is often repetitious on the surface, because it often winds back to similar themes around which his thought was currently revolving; and (2)

---

1. There were earlier attempts to articulate Langs' overall clinical theory, but they were done prior to the last phase of Langs' work. Particularly important in this regard is Raney (1984).

on the other hand, each treatment tends to be at least a little different from the last, because Langs' active and evolving thinking tends to bring him to a somewhat different understanding of the same point each time he returns to it. An obvious example of this occurs in his treatment of what he called Type One versus Type Two derivatives. In some texts, these two types of derivative communications are viewed as two aspects of the same material; in others, they are viewed as different materials altogether.[2] Langs doesn't seem to recognize that his treatment differs or trouble himself to note or correct this apparent inconsistency. Does this make a difference for understanding these two forms of derivative communication clinically? That's the sort of question we will have to ask, as we try to get to the marrow of Langs' theory. In any case, understanding both the inner dynamic of his thought and also the various ways in which it unfolds is, in my view, one of the challenges associated with outlining Langs' work as a whole, not to mention applying it. Consequently, despite this book being primarily focused on clinical practice, the chapter on Langs also amounts to an original contribution to scholarship on the clinical aspect of Robert Langs' adaptive paradigm as a whole, in part because it is the first study based on his total output.

Second, the text develops a generally underdeveloped aspect of Carl Jung's work, namely, the importance of understanding adaptation for clinical practice and technique. Especially in Jung's work *On Psychic Energy*, adaptation plays a key role, but its articulation and application are rarely touched upon, either by other texts of Jung or by Jungian authors. This is in part due to the fact that Jung uses the term "adaptation" in two different, and in some ways mutually exclusive, senses. The more common and more commonly known use of "adaptation" in Jung indicates a negative, collective mindedness on the part of the person. One meaning of "individuation" in Jung can in fact be understood as the opposite of "being adapted" (more on this in chapter 5). But there is a less known and more relevant meaning of adaptation which, far from being the opposite of the individuation process proper, is in fact a positive, individuation-directed dynamism, whose function is expressive of Jung's understanding of the unconscious psyche as a mechanism of compensation. One of the key points of chapter 4 is differentiating those two meanings of adaptation in Jung. Once that ambiguity is cleared up, Jung has a good deal to say about adaptation as a basic, dynamic feature of the psyche as well as some important points concerning adaptation very relevant to clinical practice. I will make the case that this conception in most respects adds significant material and insight into Langs' adaptive paradigm and expands the latter's value as an approach to clinical work.

Third, this study focuses as much as possible on formulating clinical principles for analytically oriented clinicians, something which especially Jungian literature often avoids, at least outside the London school. Why substantial

2. This discrepancy in Langs was first pointed out to me in conversation with Randall Hoedeman.

parts of the Jungian tradition avoid talk of clinical technique is something I also treat of and attempt to work through. The clinical principles I formulate take into account the various insights derived from both Langs and Jung and should be a worthwhile read for both Freudian and Jungian psychoanalysts and therapists.

The chapters can be outlined as follows.

The introduction poses the general problem of adaptation and clinical practice, underlining why questions associated with the nature and function of psychological adaptation constitute a significant theme. It also sketches some of the issues surrounding adaptation and clinical technique, along with the different perceptions of the value of technical studies in Freudian and Jungian thought. This approach will, it is hoped, allow the reader to understand the sometimes shared but sometimes dual context in which this book is written, in that Freudian and Jungian traditions differ on some of these issues and some of the points I underline might be responding to one rather than to the other tradition, or to both simultaneously.

Chapter 1, entitled "On Psyche and Adaptation," clarifies the notion of the psyche, the unconscious, and the picture of adaptation I am assuming. This chapter is admittedly on the borderlines of psychoanalytic theory, metapsychology, and philosophy, in that it traces some of the philosophical ideas impacting the original psychoanalytic notion of the psyche, some of which seem lost in contemporary depth psychology yet are key for understanding adaptation. In particular, it is important to understand the psyche as equivalent to the principle of organic life in the human being, at least insofar as the latter is consciously and unconsciously experienced, and to understand adaptation as therefore in part a biological concept (i.e., a concept associated with the development and, ideally, the expansion of life). Though in some measure unavoidably philosophical, I have done my best to write this chapter with the non-philosophical reader in mind and have included it mostly because the deeper sources of similarity between Langs and Jung can be missed if one does not recognize a certain philosophical similarity. Nonetheless, the non-philosophically inclined reader can in principle skip chapter 1 and still draw a good deal of what I mean to say about adaptation from the other chapters.

In chapter 2, "Adaptation in the Early Analytic Tradition," I suggest that an understanding of adaptation was both a crucial presupposition in early analytic theory but also a largely unanalyzed and underdeveloped one. In principle, Jung's *Psychological Types* is the first explicit development of adaptation, though Jung more assumes than articulates this point. This state of affairs is not due to Jung failing to recognize his book is about adaptation but rather due to the book's focus on the type problem throughout Western intellectual history. Not until the late 1930s, in Heinz Hartmann's essay on adaptation, is there an explicit, thematic essay within the depth psychological tradition consciously intended to develop a notion of adaptation. However, Hartmann's essay is more a metapsychological than a clinical text and thus we have to tease out some of its importance for our clinical considerations. The chapter concludes by making the case for the importance of Langs' contribution to psychoanalytic clinical theory with his comprehensive clinical treatment of adaptation.

Chapter 3, entitled "Robert Langs and Adaptation in Clinical Practice," offers a concentrated but largely complete picture of Langs' theory of adaptive clinical practice. As I explain in the main body of the text, I omit the study of the final writings to the extent that they focus on death anxiety, mostly because of their complexity and because, as I will suggest, they do not fundamentally change the clinical approach Langs takes. Langs' later writings, with their emphasis on evolutionary processes, different levels of psychic depth, and linkages between analytic technique and death anxiety would, in any case, require separate treatment. I also include an extended piece of a clinical case, both illustrating Langs' technical practice and showing its value for understanding unconscious communication.

Chapter 4, "Adaptation in Carl Jung," distills two, mostly opposed meanings of "adaptation" from Jung's work. Unlike Langs, Jung has only one extended treatment of adaptation (and one abbreviated version of the same), and his usage there is quite in contrast to almost all his other references to adaptation. For this latter reason as well as because the majority of substantial references to adaptation in Jung suggest a negative "collective mindedness," it is easy to miss his perceptive and original development of adaptation in his essay "*On Psychic Energy*," as well as its potential importance for clinical theory and practice. I sift through each of these points and then offer a systematic exposition of Jung's clinical understanding of adaptation. Returning to the case illustration of chapter 4, I show how the same material that one can use for a Langsian approach to the case could be used for a Jungian approach, suggesting that Langs' techniques illuminate more than Langs realized. I suggest that Langs' understanding of the psyche is substantially impoverished in comparison to Jung's and that Langs' technical approach easily expands into the Jungian, without losing the trajectory or the main ideas that Langs already developed.

Chapter 5 is entitled "Adaptation and Clinical Technique." The chapter develops a way of understanding Langs' and Jung's points of view in a such a way that (1) their ideas can to some extent be joined into a coherent theory and (2) some clinical principles can be articulated. The first part of the chapter discusses the ambivalence toward clinical technique in the Jungian tradition. The rest of the chapter articulates ways of joining Langsian and Jungian approaches, develops clinical principles on that basis, but also underlines ways in which their approaches are not compatible. However, even in this last case I try to show how their differences can in principle be corrective of the other.

It is hoped that this book will aid psychoanalysts and analytically oriented psychotherapists in their clinical practice by helping them to recognize one important factor of clinical practice, adaptation, a factor which has been underrated in the analytic tradition, even though it has simultaneously been presupposed for it. For all of us analytically oriented mental health practitioners, clinical work is complex, demanding, and many-sided; hence any articulation of a central factor in clinical practice should aim to be helpful in a practical way. The goal of this book therefore is to give both an overall sense of how adaptation has always lurked below the surface of psychoanalytic clinical theory as well as offering some practical guidance on how to recognize its impact in one's own clinical practice, with the help of two outstanding theoreticians and practitioners, Robert Langs and Carl Jung.

Note on language: A few notes on my use of language. Following Langs, I will use the terms "therapy" and "analysis" (and their cognates, e.g., "therapist" and "analyst") interchangeably, not because I think there is potentially no difference between them, but because anything I speak about in this study would appear to apply equally to each. Also, in the main body of the text, I will use the traditional "we" when referring to things previously stated in the text, since presumably both the reader and I are aware of them. When referring to my actions for example in case material, personal anecdotes, or to my correspondence with Langs, I will use "I" since it refers to my experience alone.

Introduction

Let's begin by asking the fundamental question: why adaptation? Why think, for example, that adaptation is so important for understanding clinical practice and technique? Or asked colloquially, what's so special about adaptation? Perhaps an anecdote would be the best first step toward an answer to this question.

I recall attending a case colloquium some years ago. The presenter began with a few details concerning the patient, mostly purely factual characteristics about the process (e.g., how many sessions the therapist had seen the patient), and then turned immediately to telling a dream. The dream was short and written up in perhaps three lines of text, including one major image—a bull. A couple of associations were given, but no context was offered, either (1) for why the dream might have been dreamed, (2) for why the dream might have been brought up at that point in session, or (3) why the dream might have been brought up at that point in treatment generally. The presenter, apparently at the behest of the analyst facilitator, offered only this material and immediately opened the floor for comments: the dream and the somewhat intellectualized associations, along with the general factual information, were offered as the material for the case.

At the time, I asked myself how these scant clues were supposed to reveal a patient's psychological life, a question others may also have been asking themselves given the longish pause that followed. I also felt a growing irritation in this ensuing silence. This was not the first (or the last) time that I would attend a case presentation of this kind: little more than a dream or other fantasy material with little context, a few more or less valuable associations, and some largely external facts. After the gap of silence, someone finally raised his hand and discoursed briefly on the use of bulls in the ancient Rites of Mithras, nodding as if these stories obviously amplified the image in the dream. My irritation intensified at those comments. I didn't say anything to anyone at that moment but entered my own interiority, as I tried to understand what was going on inside me.

At a certain moment, I understood at least some of my reaction: I had begun studying Robert Langs' texts just a couple months earlier and my reaction had evidently arisen from their impact. Langs' notion of what he terms the "adaptive context" grew out of his experience of supervising similar case presentations, cases where concrete events and thus concrete adaptive problems were missing. For example, the dream images by themselves were offered as clinical material. Images, as Jung indicates in many places, are the *form* in which psychic and especially unconscious material is given; that much could be granted. However, Jung also mentions in countless formulations that images are intrinsically multivalent (i.e., that they imply

1

multiple meanings and potentialities, especially when they are conceived teleologically and/or archetypally). Consequently, for us to know which of the image's many potentials are relevant to this specific patient and this specific time, it is key to know material beyond the image. We need to know, for example, some concrete (and typically current adaptive) problems to discern which of these many possible meanings most appropriately applies to this patient's experience.

Though my irritation intensified when my peer brought in the Rites of Mithras, in another way I couldn't blame him for doing it: what can one do with the presentation of an image without current activating life events or experiences, or emotionally founded associations, or early life experiences, or anything else concrete, other than turn to archetypal amplifications? And yet, though that move might be understandable, there is still the issue of *which* archetypal material to turn to. Why assume the Rites of Mithras to be a good way to amplify the bull image archetypally? Why not astrological myths associated with Taurus? Why not the story of Zeus and Europa? Why not the tradition of bullfighting? What if the Chicago Bulls loom large in the patient's psyche? What if she always experienced her father as a "bullshitter"? What if she typically felt like "a bull in a china shop"? Though archetypal material can certainly amplify the images, understanding and approximating *which* archetypal material is relevant (or at least most relevant) in any given clinical context seems to require stepping outside the image, toward what the image at least might have reference to (i.e., to the events and the psychic disturbances in the patient's life to which the patient is adapting, on which we can assume the images are commenting).

How then does one link the image to the more concrete stuff in clinical material? What relates the concrete incidents to the forms and images by which the psyche meaningfully organizes them? Classical analysis, both Freudian and Jungian, seems to have clear and valid answers to that question. For classical Freudian theory, it is by linking the images to unresolved early life experiences, experiences which cause disruptions in later conscious life to the extent that they are unresolved—the so-called reductive method. Jung for his part added to the reductive method a synthetic method, whereby the image is interpreted in terms of future possibility and future resolutions to current psychic conflict. Though Freud's and Jung's views here are in certain respects opposites, one thing they share is the assumption that something outside the explicit image is required for understanding how the image confers its meaning on concrete material: both causal-historical (Freudian) and teleological-synthetic (Jungian) construals amount to relating psychic images to potential reasons for how and why the psyche uses those images, reasons which are motivated by historical life-events or future historical possibilities.[1] The image without such concretizing reasons carries potential, but

---

1. In *Memories, Dreams, and Reflections* (Jung, 1983), Jung highlights history as one of the key features that defines analysis. For example, see the opening paragraphs of his famous chapter entitled "Confrontation with the Unconscious."

discerning which potentials are relevant requires a second, motivating factor beyond the image itself.

Hence, the experience of this presentation helped to crystalize in my own mind an important point: understanding clinical material is not simply about the images and the contents those images form; it is also about the reasons those images were formed—an essential part of analytic theory yet forgotten in the case presentation mentioned previously. Otherwise put, psychic life and the inner events which make it up are always motivated occurrences: they do not just happen spontaneously, even if they are sometimes *experienced* that way as, for example, when the motivation is still unconscious. In practice, to the extent we can find no motivation for psychic experiences and correlating images, they are either of no use for analysis or, if they have some use in principle, we cannot see what precisely that use might be. If a patient says, "I am in a bad mood, but I don't know why," we might well try to discover why—that is, what is motivating the mood and how does that motive relate to the mood? And if we find no motivation for it, one of two options seems to be the case: either it is a spontaneous but unmotivated feeling about which we can do little analytically or it *is* motivated, in which case we seek what concrete events or factors motivate the mood and what correlating images confer meaning upon the mood. Similarly, with a dream or fantasy image: insofar as we can see that image as a motivated and purposeful production of the psyche, we can do something with it analytically. But if not, we are left with a series of open questions about its meaning. The image might suggest any number of possible meanings and potentials, but without understanding or at least speculating upon the motivation the psyche had in producing it, we cannot move beyond the possibilities to its actual and specific meaning.

Though the previous discussion is an example from my own experience, it is clear that Langs had similar experiences in his supervisory groups. In the hundreds of published pages of Langs' supervisory transcripts, we see time and again that he contrasts standard, classical psychodynamics to his own adaptive approach, precisely on the grounds that classical psychoanalytic theory does not sufficiently appreciate the adaptive contexts which motivate the clinical material. Langs' formulations of these issues might have their own problems, such as his assumption that classical psychodynamics is a purely intrapsychic undertaking—an analysis of psychological material from a purely internal standpoint—which never transcends to "external," adaptive factors. While that interpretation of traditional psychoanalytic theory seems to me questionable (a point I will take up in chapter 3), it can at least illuminate why Langs thought his approach so unique: psychological conflict, according to Langs, always pertains in some measure to how a person is living out psychic life externally, in commerce with outer, extrapsychic life. Hence any purely intrapsychic approach misses a central feature of sound psychoanalytic treatment, namely, adaptive processes and their psychological impact. In cases like my earlier example, where no significant external adaptive factors are mentioned, Langs found that one cannot move from hypothetical intrapsychic factors to the actual stuff of a patient's life.

Indeed, Langs finds adaptation so compelling because he considers it the central motive for psychic life and psychic conflict. Whether adaptation is in fact the primary or exclusive motivation for psychic life is a question I will leave open at present; clearly the analytic tradition does not concur, as my examples of classical Freudian reduction and classical Jungian teleology suggest. Nonetheless, Langs deserves credit for recognizing that psychic life is unintelligible without understanding what motivates it, whether psychic conflict, dreams, (conscious) fantasies, (unconscious) phantasies, affective eruptions, or what have you.

Returning to the presentation, the presenter did not, in my opinion, give "clinical material" properly speaking, because he presented only an image, but not its possible motivations. Hence one necessary element which constitutes clinical material proper was missing. My colleague did not, properly speaking, give an "archetypal reading" of the image either, because his "archetypal amplification" amounted to little more than his own free association to the patient's material, since no (even hypothetical) motivational justification from the patient material was given. In fact, even if his association to the Rites of Mithras had some value, say as a coun-tertransference fantasy that the presenter could not hold, we still couldn't *know* that without at least a hypothesis about the possible motivations for the dream: what issue is the dream illustrating? Or what problem is it try-ing to solve? What piece of life is being imaged this way? What event in the clinical process might be evoking it? Without these questions being asked and at least speculated on, we are all largely left to our own personal free associations.

Going back then to the original question: why is adaptation so important? Adaptation is important because it constitutes at least a central motivational category for psychically important events and conflicts, and it thus is one of the essential factors in clinical practice and process as well as in anything worthy of being called "clinical material." Whether or not we agree with Langs that adaptation is the primary driving force in the psyche, we can certainly agree that it is always one of the most important forces at work in the psyche.

Yet even if we grant that adaptation is an important motivational category for psychological life, is Langs' insistence on the importance of adaptation on target? After all, would anyone deny the value of adaptation? Is emphasizing this point anything more than a pet peeve? Is it an actual emphasis of some importance?

At times, concepts which are central to a given discipline appear so obvious, straightforward, or beyond question that they seem to require no specific investigation. It may well be that, in the worlds of depth-ori-ented psychotherapies and of psychotherapies in general, adaptation is one such concept. This is not to suggest that leading analytic thinkers and practitioners have never dealt with the notion of adaptation; on the contrary, Carl Jung, Heinz Hartmann, and, closer to our own time, Langs himself have each emphasized adaptation in their works and in various ways underlined the nature and significance of adaptation for analytic process. Yet despite these investigations, it appears to this author that the central importance of adaptation for analytic process has not yet been fully appreciated.

In one sense, adaptive issues cut to the heart of the analytic process, in that one of the chief ways we tend to define psychological health is in terms of the extent to which a patient is adapted. If a person has the psychological resources to adapt to their life situation while generally flourishing as a personality, we usually consider such a person healthy from a psychological point of view. Further, many classical types of neurosis and most cases of unconscious complexes, not to mention the famous "midlife crisis," manifest themselves first and foremost in some form of maladaptive behavior, demonstrating again just how central the notion of adaptation is for analytic process and for individuation. On the other hand, ideas concerning the nature and clinical relevance of adaptation, especially in the positive Jungian sense, appear usually to be assumed rather than developed in the literature.

One of the goals of the following study, therefore, is to (1) describe and delineate adaptation insofar as it is an element of the analytic process, and (2) elucidate how adaptation entails a certain approach to clinical technique on the part of the analyst. The goal here is neither to suggest that adaptation is the only or always the most important consideration an analytic therapist should have nor that there is necessarily only one singular style of analytic or therapeutic technique. But it is one of the aims to develop some general principles (as opposed to specific precepts) of analytic technique, based on the adaptive nature of the psyche.

Now, one of the basic differences between Jungian and Freudian traditions is that Jungians, as a rule, eschew defining much by way of clinical technique, whereas the Freudian tradition historically turns to issues of technique with some frequency. This difference is by no means accidental. Jungians, as a rule, take the movement toward individuation to be the central principle for understanding psychological life. But there seems at times to be some confusion concerning what "individuation" really means among Jungians. Though by "individuation" Jung primarily meant "wholeness" or "undividedness," there is a sense in which becoming more of an individual, in contrast to being wholly subsumed into a collective, has always also been a part of the Jungian notion of "individuation." Yet these two acceptations of "individuation" are certainly different, and their meanings are by no means coextensive. Indeed, for some people (as Jung himself points out at times), their failure to be whole consists in part in not being collectively minded enough; consider, for example, various levels of schizoid personality organization. Hence these two meanings of individuation—becoming whole and undivided versus becoming able to stand individually against the collective—are clearly two different issues, even if in many cases successful analysis achieves each. The tendency to conflate these two issues, I suggest, is an important reason for Jungian's avoiding much talk about technique.

For if by "individuation" one means "a process of becoming one's unique self" over and against a collective, any reference to "technique" can sound inimical to that process, since technique suggests a practice rooted in general (as opposed to individual) conceptions of personal psychology as well as general (and thus collective) protocols of action. The underlying anxiety here would appear to be that individuation, a process and purpose which is unique to any given person, is either necessarily or at least easily lost in favor of a more generalized mode of treatment: "technique" would then suggest the practices of a collective, which, it is inferred, must override the uniqueness of any individuation process in the patient. On these assumptions, it would only be natural to conclude that general principles of technique should be applied sparingly at best.

This anxiety is certainly not unfounded; emphasis on technique at the expense, for example, of analytic relationship or a sense for the uniqueness of each individual and each individual process could indeed blind one to what is original in any given patient and thus, quite rightly, evoke such anxiety. However, as much as such a concern merits careful consideration, it is important that the response to a one-sidedness regarding technique is not an enantiadromic leap to the opposite one-sidedness. From an analytic point of view, it does not follow from the fact that technique can be used problematically that technique is a problem. What is required is not an eschewing of meditation on clinical technique but a more careful, reflective, and balanced approach to clinical technique, one conscious of the potential tension between general technical precepts and individual treatment.

Furthermore, as we will see in chapter 4, Jung develops more than one idea of adaptation, one of which could provoke these anxieties, since it suggests a negative, collective mindedness. However, the meaning of adaptation relevant to our purposes has in essence nothing to do with this more acknowledged use of the term. In *On Psychic Energy*, Jung treats adaptation as a basic, positive dynamism of the psyche, one which, so to speak, purposively leads a person into adaptive conflicts. Predicating his thinking on the teleology of the psyche and his further assumption of the compensatory nature of the unconscious psyche, Jung argues that adaptive processes provoke the development of hitherto unconscious or underdeveloped psychic functioning. Thus, on Jung's account, adaptive processes are not only essential to the psyche but are, as it were, *meant* to manifest in psychic conflicts which in turn activate psychic energy and the development of hitherto unconscious elements of the psyche. Far from being a mere collective mindedness from which a patient must be awakened, *this* meaning of "adaptation" contributes to the individuation process in the proper sense and highlights the purposefulness of both adaptive issues and the psychic conflicts they tend to produce.[2]

Our task, then is to clarify both the meaning of adaptation in analytic process and to understand how adaptation might act as a factor in clinical technique. This will entail both a general discussion of adaptation and an articulation of two central conceptions of adaptation in the analytic tradition, that of Robert Langs and that of Carl Jung. Langs' work should thereby benefit from the richer conception of the psyche in Jung and Jungian practice should benefit from Langs' fine-tuned sense for clinical technique. This goal will further require some explication of the nature of analytic technique and some discussion of whether there could be—or should be—a specifically "Jungian" technique. The conclusion will be that issues associated with adaptation, once the latter is clearly defined and understood, are at the core of a healthy analytic process and, thus, that adaptive issues do pose significant implications for clinical technique.

---

2. My thanks to Daniel Burston for pointing out that there are more than a few parallels between Jung's notion of adaptation and that of Erikson (Erikson, 1964; Burston, 2007).

CHAPTER 1

On Psyche and Adaptation

Introduction

The nature and clinical significance of adaptation is something mental health practitioners typically take for granted, characteristically treating "being adapted" as a mark of psychological health. While it may be true that, under many circumstances, being adapted can indicate psychological health, much depends not only on the given understanding of adaptation but, even more, on what value or set of values is associated with adaptation as well as the characteristics of the environment to which one is adapting. For example, adaptation to pathological social systems hardly indicates psychological health, as well-known examples like Adolf Eichmann demonstrate.[1] Indeed, it is probably due to his recognition of widespread social pathology that Jung at times conflates "individuation" as wholeness with "individuation" as uniqueness in contrast to the collective: our modern collectives are perhaps pathological enough that to be psychologically whole in some measure implies differentiation from our society and a certain lack of adaptation, at least to its specific pathologies. In any case, for the purposes of the ensuing discussions, let's begin by offering some preliminary differentiations, though a fuller clarity can only be attained by reading the entire study.

By "adaptation" we refer, first and foremost, to a basic orientation and dynamism in the human psyche whereby one undergoes or undertakes alterations in functioning, in order the better to survive, thrive, or flourish in the context of the given environment—not excluding attempts to alter one's environment. This rough and ready definition will need to be unpacked throughout the following study, to be sure, and that unpacking will include discussions of what values we attribute to adaptation and under what conditions. At this point, however, what is key is to acknowledge adaptation as a basic dynamism of the

---

1. Naturally any analysis of Eichmann would have to go well beyond the issue of adaptation, for example by understanding the nature of psychic contagion when primitive unconscious forces have been unleashed in a society. Nonetheless, Eichmann also represents someone whose individual pathology is bound up with being all too willing to adapt to the pathologies within his society.

psyche, that human beings have an inevitable tendency to try to adapt to their environments and/or adapt their environments to themselves, both physical and human, with an eye toward surviving, thriving, and/or flourishing.

Given this focus, we are not (yet) asking whether it is a *good* thing that some specific person adapt in some specific setting. Down the road, in chapters 4 and 5, we will treat of this issue more explicitly, even if briefly, because Jung's two different uses of the term "adaptation" also indicate two different value modalities. Nonetheless, we are not yet at a point to evaluate psychologically the question of whether one *should* adapt in any given setting; we seek only to understand this basic orientation of the psyche, such that human beings attempt to adapt to their environments (and/or change their environments), and furthermore to understand what clinical relevance that fact might have.

We will begin this investigation by developing some basic theoretical assumptions, in the hopes of clarifying both the nature and the value of studying adaptation in its clinical setting, assumptions that stand at the borders of psychoanalytic theory, metapsychology, and philosophy. While the non-philosophically inclined reader may skip over this chapter and still profit from the rest of this book, there will be frequent allusions to the analyses of this chapter, making it advantageous for the reader to work through this chapter as well. We make no apologies for thinking through these more theoretical propositions since contemporary psychoanalytic theory often lacks philosophical cogency and often, when contemporary psychoanalytic theorists do use philosophy, it is used in an inadequate and non-philosophical way, to the detriment of psychoanalytic theory (Mills, 2012). Some of these assumptions might seem straightforward, though the actual use of the terms being analyzed in the literature suggests, to the contrary, that some of the insights of the early psychoanalytic theorists and practitioners have been, if not lost, at least greatly obscured. Most importantly, by the "psyche" or "soul" is meant that aspect of human nature which is closely associated with organic life (i.e., with the fact that we are living organisms, and that we experience and feel ourselves alive with greater or lesser intensity), a point which gets de-emphasized due to the excessive influence of personalistic and humanistic conceptions on later depth psychology. Though "psyche" or "soul" referred to the principle of organic life in early analytic literature and in the philosophical traditions from which the notion was borrowed (Ellenberger, 2006), the combination of (1) sedimented layers of theory through more than a century of psychoanalysis, (2) problems of translation from German into English, and (3) the focus on products of the psyche at the expense of a focus on what Jung called "the reality of the psyche," have at times, in this author's view, inhibited both a straightforward understanding of the psyche and even more importantly, a clearly delineated and differentiated experience of phenomena associated with it, such as adaptive processes. We will turn to this third point—the focus on the products versus the reality (and structure) of the psyche—in greater detail in the following as well as further on in this text, as we contrast the views of Robert Langs and Carl Jung.

The Notion of "Psyche" in Early Analytic Theory

What is the psyche? The question might seem somewhat moot: the "psyche" is, so one might think, simply another term for the "mind." And while that may be true in certain circumstances, it is equally true that trying to define the psyche through a supposed equivalence to the mind is rather like trying to define the vague through the obscure. One thing we can be relatively certain about is that the current meaning(s) of the psyche or mind in the mental health professions, especially in the United States where this is being written, is not exactly the same as it was in the early years of psychoanalysis, when the term had already gone through a century of clarification by philosophers and psychological theorists and where the context and intellectual climate in which the term was being used was primarily recent German philosophy. Even though the two great founders of psychanalysis, Freud and Jung, had significantly different conceptions of the psyche, certain basic philosophical assumptions remained the same or at least parallel. It appears to us from the standpoint of the twenty-first century that some reconsideration of this original notion of the psyche is in order.

For our purposes, it will not be necessary to trace the nuances of the varying conceptions of the psyche in the psychoanalytic traditions or to attempt to defend any specific theorist over and against another. It will only be necessary to say something about the psyche based on early analytic theorizing and on the nineteenth- and early twentieth-century philosophical traditions which helped illuminate its nature. This approach is not to distract us from the main focus of this work, adaptation, but rather to highlight it. For one of the strange conundrums of speaking about adaptation in the psychoanalytic tradition is that one would expect the topic of adaptation to be widely discussed in the analytic tradition since, as we will see and as significant theorists in the field have observed, some sense for adaptation runs all the way throughout the analytic tradition. However, in practice relatively little was said about it. The argument will be that, once we understand the early analytic tradition and how it conceived of the psyche, we will also see why the tradition didn't spend as much time on defining adaptation as one might think. Furthermore, the reason for this omission was not its lack of importance but rather because it was so essential to the conception of the psyche that it, in some ways, seemed not in need of elucidation. Nonetheless, in our own time, some elucidation is necessary.

Jung's "Basic Postulates": The Reality of the Psyche

In 1934, Jung recognized that his development of analytical psychology required a statement of some of the more properly philosophical presuppositions about the psyche. This was necessary for a number of reasons, not the least being the growing materialism of the science of the time, something which also impacted psychology and psychotherapy, such as the advent of behaviorism. Because Jung clearly saw these propositions to be philosophical, and thus beyond the scope of the empirical generalizations proper to empirical and clinical psychology, he referred to these propositions as "Basic Postulates of Analytical Psychology," the title of the essay in which they are proposed (Jung, 1934). The collection of themes as well as the arguments Jung marshals in this paper are significant, though perhaps, as a rule, not fully appreciated by non-philosophically minded readers. Essentially Jung's arguments are against the materialistic and behavioristic trends in psychology and, in order to make his arguments, he draws on ancient philosophical sources.

Perhaps the most obvious borrowing from ancient philosophy concerns the concept of "the reality of the psyche" itself. Jung's goal appears to be to articulate a robust enough account of the psyche that it does not collapse into materialistic or behaviorist assumptions, as if "psyche" is just a placeholder term for mental processes, without having a definite being of its own, that is to say a unique nature or essence such that it is not simply a function of matter. For the psyche, especially insofar as it is experienced unconsciously, can be difficult not only to fathom but actually to keep hold of intellectually: science is, after all, a conscious-level practice which assumes an objectifying attitude toward what it studies. In contrast, unconscious processes are typically experienced indirectly and in a non-objectified and perhaps non-objectifiable way. Hence, one danger of "scientific" discussions of the unconscious is that its very method tends to force unconscious processes to fall through the cracks. When the early phenomenologists articulated the principle that "every mode of being requires its own mode of knowing," they did not have unconscious processes in mind. Nonetheless, the principle applies to unconscious processes as much as to conscious processes and only a method which would not objectify unconscious processes in the manner typical of natural science could in fact yield much by way of a scientific understanding of it.

Concerning the reality of the psyche, Jung turns to arguments first systematized (if not first invented) by the great Christian philosopher and theologian, St. Augustine (ca. 354–431)—though Jung fails to mention this source. Augustine lived in a period in which certain forms of materialism (such as ancient atomism) were becoming more and more widespread. These particular forms of materialism were different from the scientific forms of materialism in our own time, to be sure, but they were nonetheless materialistic in precisely the sense that they assumed that everything that exists is either material or a derivative from matter, with the consequent tendency to reduce the soul or psyche to a form of purely material being. In his work *How Great Is the Soul?*, Augustine argues that certain properties or characteristics of the psyche exclude material properties or characteristics and vice versa. Indeed, characteristics and properties we know to be valid of one are incompatible with characteristics and properties we know of the other. Hence, whatever the soul or psyche is, Augustine argues, it cannot be constituted as a material entity, since it is characterized by properties incompatible with the nature of matter. On Augustine's account, once we understand the distinct natures of matter and psyche, we recognize that, though each mode of being might be connected in a given case—as, for example, in the human being, comprised of (at least) a body and a soul—matter and psyche are nonetheless each its own mode of being and not reducible, one to the other.

To illustrate Augustine's point in contemporary terms, physical objects are characterized, for example, by having mass and extension. But one cannot attribute these same characteristics per se to the psyche. To say one has a "four-pound resentment" or a "six-inch depression" is not only unintelligible but intrinsically absurd. Similarly, to say that one's couch is narcissistic or that a cinder block has a troubling father complex makes just as little sense, except perhaps as metaphor. Yet even more important is the reason these phrases don't make sense. According to Augustine, it is because the soul has an intrinsic nature that is different from the intrinsic nature of material entities. Hence, even if we were to argue that psyche only exists *in* physical entities—something difficult to prove, incidentally—we still cannot say that the dimension of the living, physical entity we call "psyche" is itself material.

Now this form of argumentation is not common in our own time and, in part because we too are in an age of widespread materialism and behaviorism, such arguments probably wouldn't have much of an audience—though there are substantive, contemporary, and, I would argue, cogent discussions of the soul that take up Augustine's lines of thinking quite well (e.g., Seifert, 1973; Holscher, 2016). Furthermore, even when contemporary theorists are honest enough to grant points like Augustine, they tend still to undertake mental gymnastics in order to construe the psyche as somehow "really" reducible to matter (e.g., epiphenomenalism), as if there simply could not be more contained in heaven and earth than is contained in their materialistic philosophical assumptions. Part of the reason for this state of affairs is certain bad habits of modern thinking, where one asks, "how is that possible?" prior to asking "what is the nature of this phenomenon?" Naturally, if one begins with the rigid, dogmatic assumption that anything which appears non-material must somehow be reduced to matter, Augustine's arguments won't have much purchase: if I can't explain "how?" non-material being is possible, so this line of reasoning goes, I have to deny its reality. If, however, we drop the dogmatic assumption that matter is the end-all and be-all, these arguments will appear a good deal more cogent. In that case, our goal is not to reduce the non-material to the material but try to understand the non-material on its own grounds before we ask how it is connected to matter.

Whatever one thinks of the value of such arguments, what is striking for our purposes is that Jung uses exactly these sorts of Augustinian arguments to justify the reality of the psyche, indicating, it would seem, that his intent is to posit the psyche as something real, non-material, and in principle irreducible to matter and hence having its own mode of reality. Indeed, there is little doubt that Jung holds to this position because he is constantly at pains both to show the *unity* of the soul with material reality and simultaneously its *difference from* material reality. In practice, Jung's later concept of the psychoid and his use of the alchemical image of the *unus mundus* are each meant to articulate the principle of unity, even as Jung also, for example, argues for the distinction between psychic and material forms of energy in *On Psychic Energy*, thereby simultaneously insisting on their difference (Jung, 1934).

For our purposes, Jung's defense of what we might call "psychic realism"—that is, his convictions that (1) the psyche is its own mode of reality, (2) that that mode of reality is irreducible to matter, and (3) that the psyche therefore needs to be treated on its own terms rather than as a mere function of matter—has implications for how we approach adaptation and how we approach a number of characteristics Jung and Langs attribute to the psyche—in Jung's case teleology, the nature of psychic functions, and the differences between conscious and unconscious, to name a few. For this irreducibility entails treating the psyche as something functioning according to its own nature and not attempting to reduce its functions purely to material or behavioral processes or to the purely externalist styles of observation characteristic of materialistic and/or behavioristic approaches to the psyche and so much of contemporary experimental psychological research.

For this is the meaning of "soul" or "psyche" in the philosophical traditions from which psychoanalysis (and the other psychological disciplines) differentiated themselves in the late nineteenth century: the soul or the psyche is the principle of organic life in a being; it is essentially organic life to the extent that the latter is experienced consciously and unconsciously. The psyche is thus associated first and foremost with how alive a person feels, how vital and healthy, how robustly the energy of being alive courses through the person's being. We could say that the core of psychotherapeutic practice is therefore a set of *vital values*, pertaining to the expansion and flourishing of life (Scheler, 2017; Merleau-Ponty, 2002; White, 2007). Though the psyche is always more than that set of experiences—because it is also its own mode of being—it always is, nonetheless, also something experienced. When healthy, it is typically experienced as a spontaneous source and flow of energy and, when it is not, it is often experienced as if that basic "flow" is blocked or dammed. How often people come to therapy because they just feel "stuck," an image that typically expresses how the psychic flow feels blocked in some way. Consequently, when we work clinically, our work needs to be fully attuned to our own and to the patient's experiences of life and its expansion or contraction.[2]

---

2. The idea that there is a certain set of feelings that should be understood as "vital feelings" or "feelings of life" is not, so far as I know, something one finds worked through in psychoana-

These points bear upon how we are to understand adaptation. We saw earlier that by adaptation, we mean the tendency of a living being to seek survival and, for humans in particular, to seek a maximum of flourishing within a given environment, a tendency which may entail the organism to change or, if and to the extent that the organism has the power, to change the environment (or both). Indeed, this tendency toward adaptation, as we will see, correlates substantially with what Jung means by teleology, at least insofar as the latter is experienced. However, the extent to which that tendency is both experienced and experienced with genuine potency in any given person depends on a good many factors, all of which can be psychologically significant—whether inner factors such as limits of knowledge, judgment, or courage, functional deficits, emotional struggle regarding central issues in a person's life, and the like, or outer factors pertaining to the environment, such as relationship problems, financial issues, social and cultural mores, collective values, and so forth. This point suggests that part of the challenge of psychotherapy is aiding the patient in the process of liberating this adaptive tendency and its innate movement toward wholeness and flourishing from the various ways in which it is limited, both self- and other-imposed. In a certain way, we psychotherapists are in the business of unbinding the inner Prometheus: of aiding our patients in the process of releasing the inner source of life and light that moves them toward wholeness and flourishing, over and against the various ways in which adaptive and environmental factors limit this natural trend.

On this account, then, the dynamism toward adaptation is in many respects an operationalizing of the soul's natural teleology.[3] The psyche, on Jung's account, is a reality all its own and one that has an inner and consistent impulse or teleology toward its own realization and wholeness. We will see that, once we try to understand that impulse in concrete terms, one of the ways it shows itself is in the direction of new and expansive adaptations and in a correlating tendency in the unconscious toward compensation (Jung, 1953), in the ebb and flow of movement and countermovement, all with the aim of finding a psychological balance or equilibrium. In the end, the inner *telos* of the psyche toward wholeness engenders a movement toward developing parts of the psyche with which one is in some measure uncomfortable, thus evoking adaptive issues conducive to individuation.

Understanding the "Unconscious"

It might appear an unnecessary redundancy to spend much time on the notion of the unconscious in a psychoanalytic study. However, as Mills' recent investigations show, the nature of the unconscious and how it is to be understood and accessed raises a number of thorny problems (Mills, 2014).

lytic literature. Scheler, in contrast, has worked through this specific set of feelings in a number of places and his work is highly relevant to this set of issues (Scheler, 2017; Scheler, 1973).

3. Jung explicitly understands adaptation as finalistic (teleological) in nature (Jung, 1948: para. 42).

While it is not our task to resolve such problems, it might be important to reawaken in the reader a sense for how the notion of the unconscious was engendered, in order to gain phenomenological access to it within experience.

Much of the theoretical background of psychoanalysis originates in the philosophical movement known as "German Idealism." German Idealism grew out of earlier movements such as seventeenth-century Rationalism and eighteenth-century Empiricism but, nonetheless, constitutes a historically unique form of philosophy and a unique style of approaching the mind. This approach was initiated by the great eighteenth-century philosopher Immanuel Kant and developed, over the next few decades, into an entirely new style of philosophizing. I will spend a little time on the characteristics of this style because it seems to have impacted and, in some ways, generated some of the basic clinical assumptions of depth psychology.

Beginning with the late Middle Ages, philosophers tended to analyze cognition and other mental experiences into what we might call a two-term pattern. The constituents of that pattern were the "subject," referring to the person and that person's mental acts and experiences, and the "object," that piece of the world that was understood as the reference point of those acts and experiences. Hence the language of "subject" and "object" became the typical language in which to analyze any experiences in which so-called mental acts and contents played a role. This mode of analyzing is still common today in philosophical and psychological disciplines, though it is to the credit of Langs and Jung, among others, to have recognized the limits of this older paradigm.

In contrast to this medieval paradigm, Kant noted that some experiences were not adequately described in subject-object terms, that some elements of experience seem to *irrupt into* the subject-object experience, as if from "without," and are thus not sufficiently accounted for by the subject-object analysis of experience. For example, Kant suggests, if we notice certain inviolable rules of experience, such as that material objects are necessarily experienced in space and time, we can ask what is the source of that "inviolability," that "necessity," such that we can only experience them as spatiotemporal? The object can't explain such necessity because it is an empirical object and thus can only generate inductive generalizations, not necessary principles. The subject also can't explain it because we have no experience of any constitution of space and time and, in any case, experience of our inner states is also empirical: it cannot yield inviolable necessities but only empirical generalities. Hence, Kant inferred, there must be some third term, which is in some sense outside the subject-object relationship, which contributes to, forms, or molds the experience we have of material objects. This third term (or set of third terms) Kant calls "transcendental," mostly to indicate that the origin of this "other" is outside the subject-object type of experience (Kant, 1996; White, 2008; White, 2009).

As I have argued elsewhere, Kant's discovery of this mysterious third term was difficult for him to describe, since the available philosophical concepts and theories of the time more or less took for granted an exclusively a subject-object or two-term style of analysis (White, 2009). There are times therefore when Kant refers to the transcendental realm in ways that can make it sound like something on the subject side of the subject-object relationship. At other times, it sounds as if it is "between" the subject-object relationship in some respects or even as if it encompasses the subject-object relationship.[4] Giving the best reading to Kant's ambiguities, I think we can say that Kant attempts to describe an experience which philosophical theories of his time could not adequately describe, in which some third term originating outside the subject-object relationship is somehow and nonetheless experienced within it, requiring therefore a three-term rather than two-term sort of analysis of experience.

What is important for our purposes is not, for example, Kant's specific theses, such as the way space and time are injected into experience, but rather the *pattern of thought* by which Kant articulated it. That there are some contents of conscious, subject-object experience which do not seem to arise from the conscious subject or the object or their relationship but irrupt into the subject-object experience that is key here: a third term emerging from beyond subject and object which is simultaneously a factor in conscious experiencing. This pattern of analyzing experience, derived in the Modern period from Kantian philosophy, becomes a dominant form of analysis of consciousness, soul, and experience in German-language philosophy in the nineteenth century.[5] Hence, later on, when the new form of *empirical* study of mind, psychoanalysis, comes into being, the theoretical pattern (though not necessarily the actual theses) out of which it will be developed arises from this pattern developed in German Idealism. The reason for this should be clear to any practicing analyst or depth-oriented therapist: when we come across mental contents we call "unconscious," they are usually experienced by the patient as a *disturbance* (i.e., as something which is neither wholly of the subject nor wholly of the object but which emerges, as it were, in the space in between subject and object, throwing off the patient's aims and volitional projects, their ability to act, to think clearly about the world, to attain certain goals or purposes, and of course to adapt). That empirical basis seemed to the early analytic thinkers to be adequately described in the three-term pattern of analysis drawn from Kant and from German Idealism: the unconscious

---

4. Kant's ambiguity here reverberates in Jung, who at times treats the unconscious as a third, outside the subject and object, and then, at other times, treats the unconscious as an attribute of the subject. In practice this set of ambiguities becomes more confusing in Jung, in that he sometimes conflates the three-term theory of the psyche with the two-term theory of introversion-extraversion—as if unconscious depth and introversion are necessarily connected—as in his essays on Eastern mysticism. At the same time, it should be acknowledged that, since the Middle Ages, there have been few attempts to develop an adequate language for three-term theories of the mind and even fewer that have succeeded to illuminate the phenomena in question.

5. I have "filled in the historical blank" implied in this sentence in a hitherto unpublished paper entitled "On the Philosophical Origins of the Unconscious. German Idealism and the Backgrounds of Psychoanalysis," presented at Duquesne University in January 2016.

psyche was a "third term," not wholly interpretable in subject-object terms but spontaneously emerging and irrupting into subject-object experience, at least in its effects, and often derailing subject-object experiences. It is *in* subject-object experience but not *of* it.

While it might appear to the reader that this point is only at best of philosophical interest—and perhaps of no interest to analytically oriented therapists already familiar with the notion of the unconscious—it appears to this author that even analytic practitioners too easily slip into a notion of the unconscious that assumes it to be a phenomenon exclusively of the subject side of the subject-object relationship. A part of the difficulty of working with the unconscious, as already suggested, rests with the unconscious itself, which does not fit easily into purely conscious-level categorizations, like "subject" and "object." However, the further challenge is just how difficult it is to formulate something conceived of as "mental" without simultaneously making it purely subjective. Yet the unconscious, at least as it is given phenomenologically, is not simply a subjective or subject-side experience of the subject-object relationship; it is generally experienced as something from outside the subject-object relationship which emerges within it, suggesting it is not tied exclusively to one side or the other. Here too we need to be careful not to think that if we don't know "how" the unconscious could be something other than subject or object, we need to deny that it is in fact different from subject and object.

Hence, not unlike Kant's own difficulties in formulation, analytic traditions have tended to formulate two diverse and, in certain respects, mutually exclusive conceptions of the unconscious. On the one hand, analysts pose the unconscious as if it is simply an intrinsic part of an individual psyche, an element of the "subject," as especially Freud in his topographical and structural models of the psyche does. At other times, the unconscious is posed as a third term proper, something not reducible to the subject, but emerging in the subject-object relationship without literally being of either side of that relationship, as in Jung's notion of the *unus mundus* and various notions of "collective unconscious" or, in another way, in the inherently dyadic formulations of current relational schools of psychoanalysis (e.g., Mitchell, 1988). There may be merit to each of these conceptions, but the contrasts do pose theoretical problems and potential theoretical fissures in analytic theorizing, especially because the first formulation is monadic—rooted entirely in a single subject—whereas the second permits of dyadic formulations, as in Jung's alchemical meditations in *Psychology of the Transference*. At times, these theoretical fissures between the two views seem to result in some specific theorist or school opting for one at the expense of the other, a point Mills has emphasized in some of his criticisms of relational psychoanalysis (Mills, 2012; White, 2013). When, for example, a relational theorist criticizes more classical formulations of the unconscious for assuming a "self-enclosed, Cartesian subject," they are assuming the monadic reading of the unconscious, which might not be merited in a given case, and of course is also assuming that posing yet another conscious-level construct, that of relationship, resolves all difficulties associated with the notion of the unconscious satisfactorily. While some amount of operationalizing unconscious processes in conscious-level terms is necessary for analytic styles of thought, too readily accepting their adequacy as a surrogate for the unconscious raises its own set of issues, not the least that the phenomenon of the unconscious itself can be lost. It is better theoretical style to simply admit that one is not sure what sort of onto-logical category the unconscious is than either to act like one does know or to deny the existence of the unconscious because one doesn't know. If the phenomenon speaks, our theories need to adjust accordingly. We will return to the problem of these diverse paradigms in the next section.

Going back to history, wondering about the "third term" and its nature occupied many post-Kantian philosophers associated with German Ideal-ism, not the least two major figures who directly influenced Freud and Jung, Arthur Schopenhauer and Friedrich Schelling. While these two philosophers differ on many issues, what they share is that each argued (in different ways) that some element of the third term beyond subject and object is organic life, the principle which makes one alive, associated traditionally in philosophy and early psychoanalysis with the term *soul* or *psyche*. Furthermore, for each of these philosophers, the soul or psyche names some principle of organic life in animate beings which, in the case of human beings, is experienced both consciously and unconsciously as well as underlying one's fantasy life and experiences of disturbance in conscious life.

This understanding of the psyche bears some emphasis because contem-porary English can in some way belie what German-language theorists of the time were attempting to say. In English, we tend to translate the German word for "soul" (*die Seele*) rather inadequately as "mind." The term "soul" in the German language theory of the late nineteenth and early twentieth centuries typically bore connotations associated with organic life and with cognate notions such as health, well-being, and flourishing. In English, in contrast, terms like "mind," "consciousness," and the like tend to lack those vitalistic connota-tions, being bound up—largely thanks to the Empiricist tradition—with issues of cognition and allied notions such as thinking and reasoning. This identifi-cation can be strong enough that notions like "unconscious mind" can sound downright oxymoronic in English, as if one were saying "cognition without cognition." One might speculate that one important reason cognitive forms of therapy have a good deal more influence in English-language cultures than else-where is because the English-language concept of mind is so closely and uncriti-cally associated exclusively with cognition. In contrast, in the German-language theorists of the time of Freud and Jung, soul or psyche was neither exclusively nor primarily associated with cognition, but with experiencing oneself as alive, vital, and flourishing.[6]

---

6. Ellenberger (2006) illustrates just how little the original notion of psyche pertains exclu-sively or primarily to cognition and rationality, having indeed much of the irrational about it.

If we keep these points in mind, we can better understand certain assumptions not always spelled out in the early analytic theorists. For example, would it at all seem plausible to have, as Freud did, a theory of mental life and mental conflict based on sexuality, if one were talking exclusively or primarily about mind as an organ of cognition? I would say not. But if by "mind" we mean "organic life as consciously and unconsciously experienced," a sexual theory of psychic conflict is a good deal more plausible, since sexuality is an intrinsic and experienced aspect of the organic life of mammals. Furthermore, by interpreting psyche in vital rather than cognitive terms, its spontaneity becomes more understandable: organic life functions whether we want it to or not. Many of our organic functions occur without us even being aware of it, by nature producing what we term the "unconscious" (including the "conflict-free zone" of Hartmann, 1958). The psyche functions willy-nilly and autonomously, without our volition, spontaneously producing images, thoughts, and fantasies, as well as drives, desires, and conations, quite independently of our conscious intention.

That Jung understood the psyche generally in these terms is not really in question. In his theoretical essays in *Collected Works*, volume 8, Jung frequently returns to the point that the psyche is vital energy or "life energy," an energy associated with, though not reducible to, other forms of biological energy and in principle measurable as such (e.g., Jung, 1948: para. 32). This argument should not be lost on us because it points precisely to the conception of psyche being outlined here. Further, this would suggest that the mark of psychological health is how intensely alive one is and one feels, more than it is anything else and, correlatively, what makes something "pathological" is the extent to which one's unconscious complexes and, for example, typological deficiencies block, inhibit, or decelerate the expansion of life and its experience in the patient.

A final point about the unconscious may seem a purely semantic point but is, it seems to me, a central source of confusion and thus in need of clarification. There is a substantial tendency, even among psychoanalytic practitioners, to use the term "unconscious" as if it means to be unaware of something. If we analyze this tendency into its logic, it goes something like this: to be conscious = to be aware; hence to be unconscious = to be unaware.

While that logic might appear obvious, it is not an adequate description of the original notion of the unconscious or of the historical genesis of the concept (though admittedly Freud and Jung themselves sometimes speak loosely in this way). The notion of the unconscious arises in German-language philosophy; it is used first as more than a mere modifier by Johann G. Fichte and first used extensively by the great German philosopher Friedrich Schelling, in the latter part of the eighteenth century. These philosophers in virtually no sense of the term thought the "unconscious" to be some piece of psyche bereft of awareness. It would of course be accurate enough to say that they thought unconscious processes of the psyche did not include *conscious* awareness. But the point was that the unconscious is aware *in a different way* from consciousness; indeed, the unconscious could only seem to consist in a lack of awareness if one assumes the previous premise, namely, that to be conscious = to be aware. But the philosophers in question had a decisively different view. To them, the "un-" or negation in the term "unconscious" did not negate awareness per se; it negated consciousness as the only form of awareness. Hence the "un-" in "unconscious" modifies the *kind* of awareness, that it is an awareness *not* of the conscious variety; it does not negate awareness per se. Perhaps Bollas' description of the unconscious as "the unthought known" is apt here.

Tracing the history of this set of linguistic issues would take us too far afield. At this point, it is only important that we note that, contrary to appearances perhaps, this is by no means a purely semantic issue. The unconscious for the philosophers is not an attempt to describe a lack of awareness; it is rather an attempt to articulate in symbolic terms what some of the ancients— Heraclitus, Aeschylus, Plato—referred to, using a different symbol, as the soul's *depths*. Since ancient times the soul has been construed as something which has both "surface" and "depth." Consciousness is thus understood to be mostly a surface phenomenon and the unconscious as indicating depth, that is, deeper and more difficult to describe aspects of the psyche (often bound up with the primitive forces of our animality and mammality), which are nonetheless potent forces in our conscious experience. The "unconscious" is therefore not defined by a *lack* of awareness but rather by an awareness of a different kind, one that displays characteristics associated with the metaphor of "depth": they are profound, important, often primitive from the standpoint of consciousness, but also murky and difficult to grasp.[7]

The significance of these discussions for the ensuing investigations consists in the value that both Langs and Jung place on the unconscious, the extent of which is rarely held or, in our view appreciated, in our own time (by either Freudians or Jungians). Neither Langs nor Jung, for example, will consider the unconscious a mere storehouse of repressed and denied contents or defined through some total lack of awareness, though both accept Freud's assumption that repressed and denied contents are among the contents of the unconscious (though at a relatively superficial level). For each of them in their different ways, the unconscious includes not only rejected elements of conscious life, for example, or what Jung would call "unconscious shadow," but also includes its own forms of insight, of communication, and of interaction which the skilled psychotherapist must learn to recognize. Langs' later language is quite apt here: the unconscious (or, more precisely, what Langs in his later work will call—fittingly enough— the "deep unconscious") is also a *wisdom system*. And, as a wisdom system, learning from the unconscious is learning a kind of wisdom that is all its own and that requires that one learn not only the contents and structure of it but above all its subtle language. Put loosely, that language is one of *affect*

---

7. However, it is also interesting to note that, while the ancient conception of the soul's depth included such primitive forces, it was also understood to be that which links the individual to nature and the cosmos as well as to broad social and historical movements. We can see how the ancient concept of "depth" thus closely parallels some of Jung's understanding of the "collective unconscious."

and *image*, a language that is not always strictly translatable into words. In any case, the concepts of the unconscious for Langs and for Jung, though very different in certain ways, assume that the unconscious is not a blind and unintelligible terrain of images and affects without awareness. It is in fact its own wisdom system with its own language and, indeed, a sort of awareness that reaches into the depths of the soul that, though not that of consciousness, is a form of awareness, nonetheless. And both would also agree that we proceed at our own risk if we choose to venture into that somewhat foreign land, without at least attempting to learn its language.

On Clinical Interaction, or How Max Scheler Was Ahead of His Time

The problem of the "third term" beyond the subject-object analysis of consciousness mentioned earlier raises a further issue of psychoanalytic theory deeply relevant to the problem adaptation, namely, the nature of clinical interaction. Both Langs and Jung were ahead of most of their respective colleagues when it came to articulating new paradigms of clinical interaction, but the direction in which both moved was already presaged in the work of a phenomenological philosopher, one whose work can help us understand the relevant issues and possibly move us beyond the current understanding of clinical interaction.

Max Scheler was perhaps the first major philosopher to deal directly with Freud's thought and with the new study of the psyche initiated by psychoanalysis (e.g., in his critique of Freud's theory of love in *On the Nature of Sympathy* [Scheler, 2017]). In fact, even when Scheler does not deal directly with psychoanalysis, many of his critical concerns overlap with the basic phenomena with which psychoanalytic clinical theory and practice are concerned, because much of Scheler's work is a philosophical anthropology, whereby he attempts to articulate a phenomenologically based theory of human nature in general and of the human psyche in particular. Scheler's name and work was certainly known to Jung, who refers to Scheler here and there. However, the value of Scheler's work for psychoanalytic clinical theory is still a lode waiting to be mined.

Psychoanalytic clinical theory hinges on two central assumptions: (1) some specific understanding of the nature of the soul or psyche and (2) a theory of how two psyches—in this case the psyche of the analyst and that of the patient or analysand—interact with each other, especially within analytic sessions. Virtually every element of psychoanalytic clinical theory and every development of clinical technique derive from the specific formulations of these two assumptions. Accordingly, psychoanalytic clinical theory has, over the years, developed a specific language and set of concepts to describe the often subtle and at times obscure elements of clinical interaction. Yet, however valuable psychoanalytic language and its concomitant concepts are in practice, there is a certain lack of philosophical clarity in some of the central notions of psychoanalytic clinical theory, in part due to a confusion concerning which element or stratum of the "mind" we are speaking of when we talk of the psyche. It is precisely at this point that Scheler can contribute a good deal to psychoanalytic clinical theory, because he recognizes some of these central confusions and offers phenomenologically rigorous analyses to clarify them. In the following, we attempt to develop some rudimentary philosophical understanding of clinical interaction, with the help of Scheler's understanding of the "knowledge of other minds." In particular, we will draw attention to the interactive quality of psychoanalytic work and utilize Scheler's pioneering work on interpersonal psychic experience in order to develop a philosophically rudimentary but theoretically adequate description of clinical interaction.

Psychoanalytic theory originated at an intellectually interesting time, near the end of the nineteenth century. The development of an empirical psychology relatively independent of philosophy was at this point fairly recent, stretching back scarcely twenty years into the 1870s. This transformation of psychology from a more properly *a priori* discipline to an empirical one raised a number of methodological questions, such as whether psychology could be understood and articulated on the model of natural science. As time went on, Freud and Jung each in their own way recognized that any "science" of clinical psychology would at least not be a natural science in the usual sense because it required understanding phenomena outside the domain of the natural sciences, such as the concrete history of a patient as well as the range of the patient's dream and fantasy life, phenomena which entailed an expansion of psychoanalytic theory beyond exclusively natural scientific models into areas of knowledge dominated by the social and historical sciences.

Though these early psychoanalytic pioneers in some measure recognized the originality of their new discipline, it nonetheless took some time for psychoanalytic practitioners to break out of older conceptions of cognition, science, and human interaction, those based on nineteenth-century models from which the new empirical discipline of psychology arose. In the early days of psychoanalysis, for example, it was commonly assumed that the analyst was something like a neutral, objective observer of the patient, in some way parallel to the image of the objectively minded natural scientist, measuring some non-personal, material object of study. Only after some decades of practice and reflection did psychoanalysts draw a different picture about psychoanalytic practice, one in which the ideal of a totally neutral objectivity on the part of the analyst was abandoned. Put in more modern language, over the decades, psychoanalysts of both the Freudian and Jungian varieties recognized that analysts are "participant-observers" in a process (Grotstein, 1984), alongside their patients. It is particularly to Jung's credit that he seems to have recognized this prior to the Freudian tradition, in the 1930s and 1940s, though this recognition was obscured by the fact that his most perceptive analyses of these issues were posed in treatises offering psychological interpretations of alchemical symbolism, making the insight difficult to understand and, for those unschooled in Renaissance and post-Renaissance literary styles, difficult to read. By the late 1960s, Freudian clinical theory had also moved from the model of the objective analyst to an interactive model (i.e., a model where each member of the clinical dyad is in fact in an adaptive process with respect to the other member). The primary difference between them is that the analyst is supposed to recognize the fact that clinical interaction is always a case of mutual adaptation and thus draw clinical insights for the patient based on this state of affairs and based on the sources of experience, theory, and evidence that the analyst presumably has in hand.

Though this move to a more interactive and interpersonal interpretation of the clinical situation was certainly a step in the right theoretical direction, it posed an entirely new set of conundrums for psychoanalytic theoretical language, especially the language of clinical technique. This was so because the older clinical concepts used to understand and theorize about clinical experience were derived from the older, quasi-natural-scientific model of the objective observer. For example, the older model of an observing analyst relating to a patient is, of course, the familiar "subject-object" situation that defines—not to say burdens—much of epistemological theory from the late medieval period into the late modern period. On this model, subject and object are typically understood as two separate entities related basically through an external relationship, one of cognition or of acts—such as understanding, feeling, and the like—which make reference to the other party in the dyad.

A typical case of this sort of theorizing would be, for example, the classical articulation of the transference, which was understood as a kind of displacement of earlier life experience on the current experience in therapy.[8] Using the subject-object model as its basis, the classical statement of the transference would be that some psychic content—say an activated mother complex—present in the patient is "displaced" or, in other words, mistakenly experienced and attributed to the current analyst, with all the feelings, conflicts, resentments, and so forth the patient feels toward the mother now being experienced as if they actually do and ought to refer to the analyst. On this model, the patient in some way deceives themselves experientially and, ideally, the work of analysis consists in recognizing this deceptive and partially illusory experience by bringing to conscious recognition that the analyst is not the proper object of these experiences and that the root of this experience is the unresolved problems associated with the maternal object.

---

8. It is more typical of Jungians, Kleinians, and perhaps also of contemporary Freudians to understand the transference in terms of projection rather than displacement. The classical articulation of the transference, however, would appear to be based on displacement, strictly speaking, i.e., on an earlier life experience being relived in present—an experience that could of course include a projection from earlier life (Greenson, 1967).

Many of the basic, classical doctrines of psychoanalysis move along a similar axis to this example of the transference where—on the classical model—the patient is viewed in terms of being a subject with divergent and often conflicted psychic experiences, a divergence and conflict expressed with the tension between "conscious" and "unconscious" contents, and where some psychological content is interpreted as experienced, displaced, or projected onto the analyst. It is then the analyst's job to "analyze" the elements of the experience which appear to be unconscious or, in other words, unresolved and affectively overcharged or undercharged. Whether we speak of classical examples of so-called psychic mechanisms, such as displacement and projection, or psychological defenses such as denial and repression, or characterizations of psychic drives, the classical statements of these phenomena are all given in terms of a singular person, the patient, whose psyche defends, projects, displaces, and so forth in the direction of what is either the proper object or the surrogate object of such experiences, namely, the analyst. Similarly, classically formulated experiences in the opposite direction, from the analyst to the patient, are also typically put in the same terms, such as the so-called countertransference, which is basically the same transference phenomenon described previously, but from the analyst (subject) to the patient (object).

In practice, therefore, classical clinical theory and language are basically modifications of the traditional subject-object model of experience, derived from the late medieval period; it is only a more complex model because there are, functionally, two subjects and two objects, each subject referring to the other as an object. This should strike us as interesting and perhaps a little baffling, given the point outlined earlier that, in practice, the unconscious is a "third term" outside the subject-object relation. But of course, also as noted earlier, the difficulty of formulating that third term has often led both philosophers and psychoanalytic theorists to reduce the third term to some dimensions of the subject. The classical understanding of clinical interaction is a case in point.

An implicit assumption in this understanding also needs to be made explicit: among its assumptions is that experiences are basically internal phenomena which, it is true, might be characterized by what the phenomenologists call an "intentionality," but which nonetheless are understood as entirely internal *experiences*, with a superadded but purely mental reference to the object. That is to say, the subject-object analysis of the analytic experience treats the "object" as a kind of external reference point to purely internal experience on the part of the "subject."

This latter point deserves some emphasis. It is of some importance that we notice that this model, at rock bottom, takes for granted that psychologically relevant experience is essentially an *individual* phenomenon and a purely *private* affair. Indeed, it is so individual and private that, at least in the original and more classical version of psychoanalysis, one understands the inner life of the other primarily through the patient's *verbalization* of inner life. In fact, much of early psychoanalytic clinical theory is simultaneously a philosophy of language (think of Freud's theory of jokes, by way of example), because the analyst is often trying to "catch" the clues to the purportedly private and wholly internal life of the patient in the latter's discourse (e.g., through derivative communication). While language is certainly one of the key sources of our knowledge of psychic life, the emphasis on language, it would seem, hinges on the assumption that psychic life is so individual and private that language is essentially one's only more or less certain access to another's inner life, a point we will return to as we treat of Langs' clinical theory.

Though there is a certain rigor and clarity to such a picture, the many decades of analytic experience altered the picture of the psychoanalytic clinical relationship. This change is in part due to phenomena that are perhaps not usually considered by philosophers, but which are in fact quite common in psychoanalytic practice. Let's take as an example a patient experiencing some profound affect around some painful memories, traumas, or the like. At a certain point in treatment the patient, who has habitually defended against the memory and affect surrounding these events, may not quite allow themselves to fully feel the pain. At that moment, the patient's defenses re-emerge, at which point the analyst then seems to feel the patient's pain, as it were, for them. It is as if the pain of which the patient is in denial gets deposited into the analyst, who experiences some level of the patient's suffering which the patient cannot yet endure.

This latter is a dramatic and relatively intense example of a usually more common and nuanced phenomenon—one which incidentally Scheler was clearly aware of, for example in his discussion of grieving parents of a deceased child having not only each their own individual grief but also having a *shared* grief, an interactively constituted grief (Scheler, 2017). It is such experiences as these which helped to move psychoanalysis out of the nineteenth-century subject-object paradigm to a more complex, interactive model, where some experiences might be individual, other experiences might be shared, and still others might be such that one experiences another's experience before the other does—a purely interactive phenomenon. The phenomenology of these experiences more or less forced an interactive model on the theory of the clinical dyad and on the understanding of the living relationship within the dyad.

Despite this recognition of the interactive nature of clinical experiences, the earlier subject-object language and terminology remains present in both Freudian and Jungian psychoanalysis, even as both traditions have in fact moved away from the subject-object model to a more interactive model, such as one finds in relational psychoanalysis or in Jung's *Psychology of the Transference*. And, as the examples of shared experiences (as where the analyst experiences what one would expect to be on the patient side of the experience), the older model with its assumptions about exclusively individual and private experiences won't work logically. The older model assumes experience to be private, individual, and straightforwardly connected to an inner psychic experience or a projected outer experience;

hence it cannot accommodate the interactive phenomenon such that experiences may not be quite so isomorphically related to a single psyche or so private and individual as the theory suggests. Nonetheless, while the use of subject-object models is not actually coherent with an interactive model, it would be difficult simply to change from the older terminology, for a number of reasons.

First of all, psychoanalysis as a discipline is close enough to its foundational figures that the latter still loom large in all its theorizing and self-understanding. Virtually all the classical figures of both Freudian and Jungian analysis prior to the 1960s still used the older terminology and, given that in many cases they are still authorities, the older terminology, and the language game of which it is a part, is going to remain in use. Further, the role of theory in psychoanalysis is of course different from, say, the role of theory and theoretical understanding in philosophy. Psychoanalytic theory, even in its most complex, is still deeply bound up with a *practice*, namely, the practice of clinical psychoanalysis (Hartmann, 1958). The importance of this point is that theory in the psychoanalytic tradition is measured more in terms of its function and utility than in terms of its exactitude or unqualified truth. One might almost say that psychoanalytic theory is viewed as "true enough" if it functions adequately for clinical purposes. It therefore troubles your average psychoanalyst a good deal less than it might your average philosopher that this incoherence obtains.

Still, though psychoanalysts might not be troubled by this incoherence, there is perhaps more to this story. As a matter of principle, psychoanalysis generally has too undifferentiated a notion of the mind to accommodate the range of phenomena that it seeks to articulate and explain, something which we will see as we proceed to discuss Langs and Jung. The unconscious assumption lurking behind much of classical Freudian and Jungian thought is that when we talk about the soul or the psyche or what often gets translated simply as "mind," we are speaking of a uniform entity, a non-physical but almost thing-like substance with certain functions and contents, that can be defined clearly enough to be traced back to that singular entity, the psyche. But of course, on that model, it is difficult to develop the more interactive type of experience which a more contemporary psychoanalysis would want to describe, where experiences are not so bound to the individual who may originate them and where clinical experience is more like a field of phenomena "between" the members of the analytic dyad than a purely personal and private affair.

Hence it could well be that this incoherence has not been sufficiently treated of theoretically, in part because the underlying philosophical images and assumptions of classical psychoanalytic theory are inadequate for resolving the theoretical problem. While there might be practical, textual reasons for keeping the older terminology alive, there may also be theoretical conundrums that make it more or less impossible to resolve the incoherence in those terms. Yet a careful look at Scheler's understanding of some of these issues can give us at least some theoretical clarity where classical psychoanalytic theory cannot.

Understanding Scheler's notion of the soul or psyche requires some clarification beyond the language typically used by mental health professionals and often by philosophers in our time. The primary reason for this was mentioned earlier, namely, that "mind" often has a relatively thin and basically cognitive overtone in contemporary American mental health settings, especially since the advent of cognitive therapies in the 1970s and 1980s. In contrast, psychoanalysis, as we have seen, borrows its notion of soul or psyche from nineteenth-century German philosophy, where the soul or psyche is understood primarily as the principle of organic life within a living being, quite similar to the usage of soul or *anima* in ancient and medieval philosophy as well. The psyche, therefore, is not bound up exclusively or primarily with cognition but is fundamentally the principle of organic life in the human being, insofar as the latter is experienced. The psyche aims at its own flourishing or, in other words, at the expansion of life. The various functions attributed to the psyche therefore are healthy and active, insofar as they serve this function.

Scheler's notion of the psyche falls in line with this tradition, but also requires somewhat more differentiation. Within the stream of human experience, Scheler distinguishes three diverse sources or centers of activity: the person, the psyche, and the lived body. Each of these centers has a distinctive and correlating form of activity, what I have called elsewhere Scheler's "tripartite anthropology" (White, 2001; White, 2014). For example, following his analysis in the *Formalism* (Scheler, 1973), Scheler calls the activities characteristic of the person "spiritual acts" and "directions" (the latter term referring habits, such as developed virtues and vices). "Spiritual" here does not have any quasi-religious overtones, as it often does in English, but translates the German *geistlich*, which indicates a specific, non-physical mode of being (Scheler, 1973; White, 2001; White, 2014). These spiritual activities of the person are contrasted to the activities of the soul or psyche, which are termed "functions," and which possess their own form of functional or operative intentionality, in contrast to the act-intentionality of the person. Acts, on Scheler's account, arise from a kind of a voluntary sovereignty which a person has over the execution of his or her acts and spiritual being. In contrast, psychic functions tend to arise spontaneously and autonomously, unless the spiritual person intentionally inhibits that function or functional expression, by acts such as conscious suppression. Thus, according to Scheler, the dimension of experience we might call "spiritual" or personal and that which we might call "psychic" or "psychological" are different, the former relating to what makes human beings distinctly personal, the latter more related to what makes human beings mammalian animals. Scheler's discussion of these issues is in some sense a common theme among German and Middle European philosophers in the first half of the twentieth century (including

Edmund Husserl and Ernst Cassirer, for example), where the connections of and the distinction between spirit and life were widely discussed.

Scheler further distinguishes lived body experiences from those associated with either spirit and psyche, by virtue of their essentially bodily character, of the relative passivity of the conscious subject with respect to them, and above all a lack of intentionality proper (in the phenomenological sense of "intentionality"). Lived body experiences include sensations, the sense of being localized in (physical) time and space, and other experiences that have both the vector of physicality but also that of being experienced as one's own. For Scheler, lived body experience is not properly a "consciousness of" anything but rather a bodily awareness of experiences largely passively undergone. Lived body experiences, as an experience purely immanent to the consciously lived body, condition the awareness of sensuous experiences and explain why they are experienced as *my* experiences.

Though, according to this account, there are these three distinct centers of experienced activity, the activities of each tend to interweave with the others throughout the totality of experience and mental activities. Indeed, many sorts of activities are actually multi-layered experiences comprising activities of two or all three of these centers. One example that Scheler analyzes in both the *Formalism* and *Sympathy* is what he terms "vital sympathy," an activity which requires simultaneously the experiences of vital identification—identification with a living other at the level of psyche or soul—and spiritual differentiation, that is, the cognitive recognition that that with which I am identifying is not in fact mine (White, 2005; White, 2012; White, 2014). Thus, human experience for Scheler can be understood to be many-layered and multi-faceted and to require for their analysis more than a simple isomorphic analysis of subject and object.

We have spent some time on this differentiation because we believe it is often missed in discussions of Scheler, including by competent thinkers. Alfred Schütz, for example, criticizes purported inconsistencies in Scheler's account of the mind, yet the inconsistencies he points to seem relatively easily resolved once one recognizes Scheler's differentiation between the spiritual and personal element of experience, on the one hand, and its psychic dimension, on the other. In any case, for our purposes what is important is that the psyche, on Scheler's account, is not the totality of all that might be deemed "mental," but is rather the principle of organic life and also, to the extent psyche is experienced, the basis of "consciousness" in the narrow sense, as well as the basis of what psychoanalysts term "the unconscious." This depth is not always present to consciousness but nonetheless can impact conscious experiences. Hence psychology, according to Scheler, is primarily the study of the psyche or soul and its functions, in contrast to that part of "mental" experience which is personal and spiritual, which is the proper domain of phenomenology alone. If by "mind," we mean the full range of human experiencing and acting, then according to Scheler only one sector of that full range is the proper domain of psychology and thus of disciplines like psychoanalysis: the sector referring to psychic life and functions. The latter pertain primarily to conscious and unconscious experiences associated with the psyche, the experience of organic life, and only indirectly to the domain of experience inherent to either spiritual or lived body experiences per se.

With these differentiations in hand, we can better understand the remarkable final section of Scheler's book on *Sympathy* and its immediate relevance to the issue of clinical interaction. There Scheler is concerned with the sorts of experiences that particularly pertain to the interaction of human beings *at a psychic level*—a point we emphasize because it does not come through as clearly in the English translation as it might, since the translator uses the word "mental" rather than "psychic" when referring to psychic functions. There might be good reasons for the translator's decision, not the least that "psychic" in English can refer to what are conceived of as preternatural powers of the soul, something of which Scheler is definitely not speaking. Nonetheless, this element of the translation seems to undermine the specifics of the difference between spirit and psyche in Scheler: both spirit and psyche are in some sense "mental."

Two assumptions that Scheler developed first in *Formalism* are brought to bear on the problem of the knowledge of other minds in *Sympathy*.

(1) First, Scheler makes clear that the question of the knowledge of other minds is not a question to be posed concerning that dimension of the human being we have termed spirit or person. On Scheler's account in *Formalism*, the spiritual person is in fact a wholly private dimension of the human being. Indeed, in principle, the only two ways one knows a person *as* a person is either by virtue of revelation (i.e., by means of a person communicating experiences to another) or second by the attempt to recreate and reproduce (e.g., imaginatively) in one's own spiritual being what has been lived by another. Here, in fact, the knowledge of other minds is always indirect, either through communication or through the reproduction of another's acts.

(2) The second assumption concerns the psyche. On Scheler's account, the psyche or, as we could say, the psychic dimension of experience is not private but rather expresses itself automatically. That is to say, the psyche is not like the spirit, the latter being subject to a kind of voluntariness on the part of the person. Psyche is rather relatively autonomous in its functioning, and it is by nature expressive and expressing itself. We can of course modify both what and the extent to which the psyche expresses itself by means of certain spiritual acts, such as suppression. But that is always an interruption of the natural process, because the psyche left to itself expresses its inner life, at least to some extent, outwardly. Indeed, this element of Scheler's teaching does not fundamentally change to the end of his life (e.g., in *Man's Place in the Cosmos* [Scheler, 1981], where he defines life in general—and psyche in particular—in part through its expressiveness). In this respect, there is a certain parallel between spirit and lived body for Scheler, because lived body experiences, such as pain, also cannot

be co-experienced by another, though for different reasons than spirit; only psychic functioning can be co-experienced with another.

We should notice that from the outset Scheler's differentiation between spirit and psyche virtually poses an objection to the version of psyche present in classical psychoanalysis. I noted earlier that the psychoanalysts tend to treat the psyche as the single source of so-called mental experience, whereas Scheler differentiates three sources of such experience. Furthermore, the older model of psyche in psychoanalysis interprets the latter as a largely self-enclosed, private sphere, largely known through verbal communication on the part of the patient. According to Scheler, in contrast, such an analysis contradicts the nature of psyche by conflating essential characteristics of the personal *spirit*, such as privacy and individuality, with that of the *psyche*, which not only is not private but which by nature expresses itself outwardly. The spiritual person is by nature private and known only through revelation; the psyche, by contrast, essentially expresses itself and is thus a far cry from a self-enclosed mental system.

In this final section of *Sympathy*, in fact, Scheler makes one of his most controversial claims, one whose very sense seems rarely appreciated, in part because interpreters do not adequately differentiate spirit and psyche. Scheler's claim is that the psychic life of the other is in principle experientially just as open to us as our own psychic life and, further, that both are known through one's "inner perception."[9] While this claim might seem controversial at first glance, we should not be entirely surprised that Scheler thinks that we have an unusually high level of awareness of another's psychic life: short of any of us consciously suppressing the expressivity of psyche, the psyche expresses itself outwardly by nature. Indeed, looking directly to the experience one has as an analyst, none of this should come as a surprise. Who among us who are analysts does not recognize the extent to which we are reading our patients' psyches through their body language, facial expression, and movements just as much as by their expressive language? Any conscientious analyst, as is well known, recognizes the extent to which psychic life is characteristically expressed, to the point that we often have at least a general idea of what's going on in our patients' lives as they walk into the office and before their words confirm it, just from "reading" their various expressions. It is just this basic phenomenon that Scheler analyzes, and it plays a substantial role in our analytic work.

Indeed, Scheler's descriptions of this phenomenon expand the expressiveness of the psyche also to our central analytic tool, language. Scheler says, for example, that the psychic stream of intersubjective experience is originally undifferentiated as regards to what is mine and what is thine. For example,

---

9. Calling this experience "inner" is in contrast to the "outer" perceptions associated with sensuous experience. The term inner does not mean that the experiences are happening only "inside" the person, since inner and outer are simply vantage points from the standpoint of psychic experience.

in the midst of an intense conversation, we often do not know who originates an idea or a feeling and often cannot determine the source of ideas or feelings that we have. Something similar often happens in the midst of an analytic session—indeed, *especially* in analytic sessions, where practices connected to free association and reverie are typical to the practice. These examples elucidate the point that psychic experiences, including the affective, instinctual, conative, and imaginary elements, are, as it were, experienced *in* psychic life but often without a definite connection or clear awareness as to who originated these elements. As we know well through clinical experience, much of the liberation that occurs for our patients through the analytic process derives from working through what psychic contents—affective, ideational, or what have you—are really such that they want to "own" them and which ones not. It is evidently because of this constituted psychic stream in clinical experience that the latter in some way can be a microcosm of the life of a patient because what occurs in session will tend to have the same expressive characteristics as non-clinical experience.

To put this point perhaps more starkly, *we are by nature awash with each other's psychic lives*, whether we know it or not, and thus many psychic experiences we have may not at all originate in us. This situation is not necessarily a function of any intention on the part of any of those present; it is rather a function of the nature of the psyche which always juts beyond itself into the world, expressing some of its psychic functioning automatically and autonomously. Basic human experiences like the not understood visceral reaction we have on meeting someone for the first time, the strange feeling of expectation we sense from another, the gut feelings that seem to approve or disapprove of someone for no clear reason, would all count as pure psychic reactions which our psychic life may express and which others' psychic life may express toward us, often as a barely recognized subtext beneath our conventional politeness.

The significance of this point is manifold. For one, Scheler's claim that others' psychic life is as open to us as our own is a product of the facts that (1) the psyche naturally expresses itself and (2) we are often not clear as to which psyche the content we are thinking or feeling is attached to or originated from. The stream of experience is, so to speak, "already out there" because it is psychic expression, an expression which is originally experienced as undifferentiated in social experience. Understood in this way, we can at least see why Scheler would not think it is controversial to say that the mind of the other, insofar as we speak of the psychic level, is as open to us as our own, because we are awash with each other's psychic life from the start and because this implies a shared stream of undifferentiated experience in which any kind of ownership of psychic contents is not at first noticed or at least clear, and not achieved unless one consciously and intentionally seeks to find out who originated or who owns the specific content.

Scheler's picture therefore is of an undifferentiated psychic context in which our life occurs: in any interpersonal or social interaction, there is always a third thing that emerges, some psychic unity formed of what is being expressed on the part of the psyche of the parties involved.[10] This interpersonal stream of psychic life is not reducible to either or to all the persons involved. Further, this description and theorization of psychic life conforms better with psychoanalytic experience than available psychoanalytic theories of clinical interaction, whether the original subject-object model or later, more relationally based theories. It is standard in psychoanalytic theory to recognize that experienced psychic phenomena are often not experienced as that clearly or certainly connected to either psyche in the clinical dyad. Winnicott's notion of the "me-not-me" continuum is an example of this as well as various of the relational theories of psychoanalysis, all of which assume something like a field of experience "between," as it were, the members of the psychoanalytic dyad. Among psychoanalytic theorists, however, ideas of Freudian Thomas Ogden and Jungian August Cwik come closest to Scheler, in that they posit, beyond the individual psyches of the analytic dyad, what they call an "analytic third," a term expressing how there is a third psychic thing besides those two individual psyches in the consulting room, which seems to arise from the two members of the dyad but is not reducible to either of them. Nonetheless there is some difference because Scheler would think one's theory should *begin* with the undifferentiated sphere of psychic life, since that is what is phenomenologically given (e.g., in the experience outlined earlier of the analyst feeling the affect for the patient), rather than assume that the latter must be a theoretical epiphenomenon of two separate subjects.[11] Hence, to use Scheler for psychoanalytic theory would suggest that much of the work in a session, for example regarding transference and countertransference, is not about a purely subject-side experience of each but about the differentiation of psychic contents in a stream or field in some measure undifferentiated from the start with regard to subjects and objects and with regard to conscious and unconscious, always acknowledging the possibility that some piece of that experience is really about something original to the third, rather than analyst or patient.[12]

Indeed, this approach to psychic life highlights the weaknesses of the old subject-object model. While there certainly are experiences which can

10. Interestingly enough, this discovery of Scheler's is taken for granted in Western esoteric psychology, in the form of what is termed an "egregore" (Stavish, 2018).

11. While this theoretical difference between Scheler, on the one hand, and Ogden and Cwik, on the other, does not appear to change much from a technical standpoint, it would require some re-articulation of the analytic third. For example, Ogden (2004) suggests the analytic third arises from projective identification, thus attempting to formulate the third in terms of a prior subject-object (though unconscious) experience. Scheler would invert that order and say that the third is prior to defining subject-object sorts of experience.

12. It was because Jung recognized this problem of the undifferentiated stream of experience that he demanded future analysts be analyzed. Without the level of self-knowledge that analysis gives, it is difficult to know whose (counter)transferential contents are dominating any analytic session.

be well or at least adequately described in subject-object terms, the bulk of human experiences are not well described that way. The subject-object model is particularly helpful when one is talking about cognition in the narrow and technical sense of the term—when one recognizes some entity *as* a certain sort of entity—but is rarely adequate for other experiences where that narrow cognitive focus is not necessary. Whether one moves past innumerable unnoticed things on a walk or makes love or drives a familiar route, most of these experiences are not well described as "focusing on an object." One's vague, uninterested movement around objects or intense immersion in sexual vitality or bland familiarity with the route are all experiences but not ones in which one posits oneself as a "subject" and focuses consciously on another entity as an "object." The fact of the matter is that there is little reason to think the subject-object paradigm terribly useful for many and perhaps most experiences, at least interpersonal ones.

Further, Scheler's understanding of the original stream of psychic life can help us to understand basic psychoanalytic data potentially better than classical psychoanalytic theory. Rather than understanding, say, transference, projection, and other psychic mechanisms as a movement of psychic content from one private psyche to another, a very implausible theory in practice, Scheler begins with the proposition that the psyches of each are open, expressive, and mutually connected due to the nature of interpersonal and social experience, such that the psychic material to be analyzed in session is always potentially already available and much of it not definitely attached to one or the other psyche. Similarly, unconscious communication, the fact that one can recognize psychic processes beneath the surface of consciousness, makes more sense on such a theory, precisely because the psyche would, on Scheler's model, express such material automatically and autonomously. Scheler's theory would thereby demystify a good deal of psychoanalytic theory.

It should further be noted that, since the 1980s, there has been a great emphasis in psychoanalysis on the interactive and relational approaches to psychoanalytic clinical theory and practice, a move that as a whole seems positive. However, in practice, relational theorists still seem at times to muddle through theoretically what relationality means, in part because they often assume relationality to be something built from human individuals, rather than beginning their theorizing from an original undifferentiated stream of shared psychic experience, born of the fact that we are always expressing psychic life and thus expressing toward others, in such a way that we often don't know where our experiences or content originate from: did they originate in me or did I absorb them from someone else? Scheler's distinction between spirit and psyche and his insistence on starting with the phenomenon of psychic experiences allows him to *begin* with relationality and interaction, rather than having to build it up from two purportedly separated individuals in the analytic dyad. Further, Scheler's theory makes much clearer the fact that the "subject" of psychoanalysis is in fact *not* the whole person or the whole of a person's mental life, but just that sector of mental life associated with the psyche and refers to the other sectors, spirit and lived body, only the extent that the latter are connected to or expressive of psyche.

While this analysis of clinical interaction points to a number of areas where new questions emerge, we will have to set those aside for the moment. Suffice it to say that, on Scheler's model, we begin to see why the "third term," the unconscious, is so difficult to comprehend. For one, though one might assume the unconscious to be a subjective phenomenon, based on Scheler, we can see that in fact the subject-object analysis refers not to ontology but only to a specific cognitive and experiential *situation*, in which the conscious surface of the psyche focuses on something as its referential object. However, psychic life is hardly composed primarily of such situations, because in practice we are always forming largely unconscious psychic matrices with others which are not well-described in subject-object terms and which form an undifferentiated stream, except to the extent we try consciously to differentiate it. This analysis also expands the notion of the unconscious by recognizing that the unconscious is not essentially personal or spiritual, but is essentially vital (i.e., pertaining to us insofar as we are organic beings), and also essentially includes interpersonal and social dimensions. No glib subject-object analysis can capture the unconscious as a phenomenon and any worthwhile acknowledgment of the unconscious entails a break with the ancient subject-object model of mental life rooted in medieval philosophy. Indeed, there is good reason to think that standard ontological categories simply do not describe the unconscious well and that, in contrast, we need to mold our ontology of the mind around the unique phenomenon of the unconscious.

For our immediate context, presumably the reader can see why this introduction of Scheler is so important. There is an essential, purely psychic sense of "adaptation" which occurs in every relationship and which is generally amplified in the clinical psychoanalytic setting. That is to say, there is not only a specifically physical environment which poses an adaptive context in clinical psychoanalysis—what Langs' famously refers to as the "frame" of psychotherapy and analysis—but a distinctive *psychic environment*, which is in part the product of the mutually productive unconscious psychic factors on the parts of both patient and analyst or therapist. As we will see, Langs' outstanding contributions to understand the frame of psychotherapy and psychoanalysis nonetheless did not adequately pick up that there is a further and often more important environmental factor, namely, the largely unconsciously constituted psychological environment, the analytic third, in which the workings of all analytically oriented therapy function.[13]

---

13. See (White, forthcoming c) for other ways in which Scheler's philosophy is useful for understanding psychoanalytic ideas and theoretical assumptions.

Conclusion

While this discussion of areas associated with psychoanalytic theory, metapsychology, and philosophy might seem tangential to the clinical problem of adaptation, we have hinted that there are several ways in which these conceptions bear upon understanding adaptation. Furthermore, it is crucial that fine-tuned and specific treatments of clinical problems be understood in terms of broader theoretical presuppositions and, as will frequently come up in the ensuing investigations, many theoretical problems as well as clinical issues associated with both adaptation and clinical technique in part arise from inadequately posed theoretical assumptions. At this point, at least the following can be said regarding the three overall points in this chapter.

(1) We have emphasized an organic and dynamic conception of the psyche both because we believe it to lie at the core of psychoanalytic theory and also because it is the conception used throughout the rest of this work. The psyche, on this account, is not to be understood to be coextensive with everything we might call "mind," and it is not to be understood as essentially cognitive or necessarily associated with rationally based acts. Rather, the psyche is the vital soul, characterized by the same teleological drive for health and well-being which seems to characterize all organic beings, attempting to flourish in whatever context they happen to be. The psyche is, in other words, the spontaneous vital energy and movement in the person toward greater life and adaptation will be the primary expression of this movement. Cognition and other spiritual acts are therefore secondary to its functioning because the psyche is concerned with spiritual acts only insofar as they contribute to or inhibit the psyche's own movement toward life and its fullness.[14]

(2) Understanding the psyche in these terms is also key for understanding adaptation. For adaptation is first and foremost a vital concept, a concept born of the theory of living organisms and their relationship to their environments (Hartmann, 1958; Langs, 2004). Adaptation is the expression of the basic drive within any living being toward its own flourishing and development, as expressed in how it interacts with its immediate environment and that is true whether we speak of "adaptation" as a *process* (e.g., that process of adapting [or failing to adapt] to some environment) or whether we mean by "adaptation" a *state*, the state of being adapted (or maladapted) (Hartmann, 1958). "Adaptation," then, is a general concept referring to a living entity and its relative success, in process or state, of having a relationship to its physical and/ or non-physical environment conducive to its flourishing.

(3) For this reason, adaptation is not, for example, an auxiliary function of the psyche but a dynamism intrinsic to the nature of the psyche, because

---

14. Indeed, since cognition can have quite different purposes from helping us become and feel more alive, we can infer that cognition proper is only secondarily a psychic function. As we have argued elsewhere (White, 2001; White, 2014), cognition proper pertains to the spirit rather than psyche, even though it can also be conducive to psychic flourishing under certain circumstances.

adaptability is one condition of the existence and flourishing of organic beings (and therefore of human beings); adaptation is essential to life and its expansion. The adaptive dynamism is thus more fundamental to the psyche than psychic functions and emerges within psychic functions as one of the principles of the latter's development, as we shall see. If anything, the Jungian differentiation of fundamental attitudes (introversion and extraversion) and the four primary functional ranges (thinking, feeling, sensing, and intuiting) *specify* the more fundamental impulse to adaptation. Furthermore, though the adaptive dynamism is intrinsic to the psyche, it is not uniform in its expression in any given person: one person may be highly adaptable in feeling life but far less so in thinking life whereas for another it might be the opposite.

Beyond those valences, there is also a range of flexibility and rigidity in adaptability, both in general and according to specific functions. While "flexibility" is generally considered psychologically a positive and "rigidity" a negative, it is important to recognize that adaptation is connected to the teleology of the psyche (i.e., to a certain destiny of value realization that a person is in some sense "meant" to embody in the process of life). This teleology suggests that one can also be too flexible in one's adaptation since adaptation is meant to be at the service of the teleological direction of the psyche. Put in more traditional psychoanalytic terms, we could say that adaptation is meant to build up positive *character*, positive personality habits and tendencies (what the ethical tradition would call "virtues") that co-direct a person's ego toward what in truth fulfills the personality. There is in fact something of a dialectic between adaptability and teleology that does set limits on the proper range of adaptation in any given person. Though it would not be accurate to characterize those limits as "rigidity," free-flowing adaptation without limits is also not an ideal.

(4) These features of adaptation underline the importance of Jung's concept of the "reality of the psyche." The psyche, on this account, is a real (though non-material) principle which enlivens the human being; it is not experienced uniformly because it is comprised of a number of actual and experienced variables, among other things of adaptive valences, functional ranges, general attitudinal directions and orientations (introversion and extraversion), and complexes, all of which are in varying degrees conscious and unconscious. Consequently, the psyche is both phenomenologically given—reveals itself in the warp and woof of experience—and requires that it be treated as phenomenon *sui generis*. Understanding the psyche as an actual entity rather than a mere placeholder for the phantasy life of an individual will help underline some of what's missing in Langs' earlier conceptions of adaptation.

(5) The specifics of how adaptation works will depend on the type of organism in question and the various ways in which it can and does interact with its environment toward its own benefit. In the case of the human organism, as we will see, adaptation requires we both admit the

unconscious and its specific processes and that we recognize the unconscious not as a lack of awareness but as a specific kind of awareness, one whose own wisdom and insight must be learned at a conscious level. This further entails a central point in Langs' conception of the psyche, namely, that the unconscious psyche is not simply a series of intrapsychic images we use to resolve our problems but a mysterious yet real source of awareness and insight that is often lacking at the conscious level, unless we can consciously come to understand what it is expressing. Understanding adaptive problems and solutions clinically requires a robust and living understanding of the unconscious as a cooperating "other" in our psyche, accompanying and potentially—if appreciated—aiding each of us on our path to individuation.

(6) Finally, following both Langs and Jung, it will be necessary that we recognize adaptation not only as a general principle for understanding a patient's clinical material but especially important for understanding clinical interaction, such as the relational and transferential content that occurs in the clinical interaction. It is to both Langs' and Jung's credit that they recognized this point, though their separate understandings of the psychic interaction are, in this author's view, theoretically too weak to account for the phenomena they recognized. Indeed, once a better articulation of the "analytic third" in terms of the nature of psychic reality and its distinction from spiritual and personal acts is recognized, the nature of the interactive process comes significantly more into focus and the precise way in which clinical interaction is a mutual adaptation also comes into view.

While these are not the only reasons for discussing the three general points of this chapter, they should be sufficient for recognizing their importance. The following chapters move from the this theoretical outline to the concrete life of the psyche and its manifestation in clinical interaction.

CHAPTER 2

Adaptation in the
Early Analytic Tradition

Introduction

The concept of adaptation has a mixed history in the early analytic tradition. While it is a concept that has implicitly run throughout the major analytic traditions, it has received relatively little explicit attention, especially as a useful clinical concept. Interestingly enough, Jung can in principle be understood to be the first analytic theorist to offer a thoroughgoing analysis of adaptation, assuming one reads *Psychological Types* as describing generic forms and ranges ("types") of conscious adaptation (Jung, 1923a; Hartmann, 1958), rather than static categories of personality organization, this latter perhaps being typical of Myers-Briggs-inspired readings of the psychological types ("personality types"). In fact, Jung's earlier work, which later became *Symbols of Transformation* (Jung, 1952), can also be understood as a work either on or at least largely about adaptation, to the extent that transformation of libido (psychic energy) through compensation is one of its central threads, something we will see in part defines adaptation in Jung.

Perhaps the clearest and most definitive theoretical statement on adaptation by the early psychoanalysts doesn't appear until the late 1920s and is then revised and re-issued in 1948, Jung's *On Psychic Energy* (Jung, 1948). There were however a few other attempts in the analytic tradition prior to the 1960s to articulate theoretically the nature and value of adaptation that are worth our attention. In the following chapter, we set the stage for our understanding of Langs and Jung by examining two other major analytic authors, Sigmund Freud and Heinz Hartmann.

Sigmund Freud

Sigmund Freud assumes a concept of adaptation throughout his work, as leading authors in the psychoanalytic tradition have acknowledged (Hartmann, 1958; Rapaport and Gill, 1959; Greenson, 1967). Hartmann and Greenson agree that an adaptive point of view accompanies all the varying metapsychological views typical of classical Freudian psychoanalytic theory, such as the topographic, genetic, structural, and so forth (Hartmann, 1958; Greenson, 1967), suggesting—as did our introduction—that adaptation cuts to the heart of all psychic functioning. Nonetheless, Freud offers little by way of the development of the nature of adaptation or of its clinical relevance, resting satisfied with broad descriptions of adaptation. In fact, Freud rarely uses the term "adaptation" itself, instead describing the psyche's relationship to "reality factors," something which is synonymous with adaptation.

For example, Freud as a matter of course assumes a concept of adaptation as part of a working conception of what counts as "normal" psychology. In his classic paper, "Formulations Regarding the Two Principles of Mental Functioning" (Freud, 1911), Freud offers an extremely brief development of the notion of adaptation. Roughly speaking—and it should be noted that he acknowledged the "roughness" in the paper itself—Freud contrasts what he terms the "pleasure principle" to what he terms the "reality principle," each, as it were, competing principles of mental functioning. At this point in Freud's career, he understood pleasure-seeking (and its complement, avoiding pain) to be the primary motivating principle in the human psyche. However, Freud maintains, though the pleasure principle is the primary principle in mental life, maturation includes acknowledgment of and motivation by a secondary principle, the reality principle, which both acts as a check or limit on the range of pleasure and teaches one how to preserve more valuable and more lasting pleasures by renouncing lesser or more uncertain pleasures. Evidently, this theory is a description of what was once called the "conservation of energy," encouraging one to focus one's energy on more essential or superior pleasures, and assumes that one of the outcomes of a healthy adaptive process is that one articulates a *hierarchy* or *rank-order* of values (i.e., a conception of what counts as a superior versus inferior pleasure) and adapts accordingly.

Whatever the worth of this classic paper for understanding the psyche and mental functioning in general, it does little in the way of elucidating the nature of adaptation. In certain respects, in fact, one might say that this early paper is most important for being the "standard case" for discussions of adaptation in the Freudian tradition prior to Langs, Merton Gill, and their circle. It is not that there was no acknowledgment of adaptation in the Freudian tradition; quite the contrary, adaptation is frequently mentioned though characteristically as a side note. It is, rather, that adaptation is more or less taken for granted and thus not really developed regarding its significance. While this might seem an odd state of affairs, it is a consequence of points made in chapter 1: the psyche is understood in the early analytic tradition as the principle of organic life, and adaptation is always assumed to be one of its basic and essential characteristics. That being the case, it is understandable that adaptation is more taken for granted in early psychoanalytic literature than many other concepts relevant to psychic life. Whatever is taken to be of the essence of psychic life—and to be generally acknowledged as such—will tend simply to be assumed and not necessarily seem to be in need of articulation.

Consequently, the paper's value from the standpoint of the theory of adaptation and clinical practice is rather that it acknowledges adaptation to reality as a basic drive in the human psyche—even though it treats adaptation, implausibly, as a kind of auxiliary function to the pleasure principle. This is implausible for two reasons. First, because, as underlined in the last chapter, organic life primarily seeks its own expansion and flourishing, and does so autonomously and automatically; hence pleasure is not the primary goal of psychic life. The healthy psyche certainly seeks pleasure, but it does so *to the extent* that pleasure is experienced as expansive of life. In contrast, a person who seeks pleasure primarily—what the philosophical tradition termed a *hedonist*—is, at least in this author's view, functioning in a psychologically unhealthy way, either through ignorance of what one's genuine flourishing consists in or through pathology, since pleasure is neither the exclusive nor the primary goal of organic life.

Thus, contrary to Freud, it would appear that the "reality principle" is not just about delaying gratification, conserving energy, or discovering what pleasures appear more essential than others, but about which pleasure experiences aid one in being or at least in feeling more alive and vital. Otherwise put, the value of life and its expansion is, as a rule, experienced as higher than the value of pleasure and thus adaptation to what counts as "life expanding" can be and, in a healthy person, generally is experienced as a superior motivation to physical pleasure. In contrast to Freud's analysis, it appears that people often sacrifice certain pleasures not only for greater pleasures but more often and more importantly for values they experience as altogether higher than pleasure—a difference not merely of degree or intensity, but a difference of kind. Indeed, if that were not the case, it is difficult to see how any classical description of the sublimation of psychic energy could be conceived of as psychologically healthy or worthwhile. Hence, though Freud correctly notes a kind of value hierarchy, such that the reality principle forces one to consider what pleasures are superior or inferior—characteristically hierarchical thinking—he does not, it seems, correctly analyze what the hierarchy consists in.[1]

---

1. The full argument for this point would also require some analysis of the various meanings of "pleasure." Scheler (1973) develops the differences between bodily pleasure and feelings of life, vitality, and well-being.

The second reason this thesis seems implausible is that pleasure is often—indeed typically—a secondary experience based on a prior experience of (higher) value. Freud's understanding of pleasure evidently refers to "lived body" experiences (i.e., the body insofar as it is "lived in" and experienced). While such bodily pleasures are certainly important in life, they are often mediated through other experiences of value. This is especially obvious in some aesthetic experiences, such as the experience of beauty. The sunset one delights in is first and foremost an *emotional* response before it is experienced also as a kind of bodily pleasure, resonating throughout the body with the wholesome sense of life and its wonder. Furthermore, were one to aim at that bodily resonance and wonder without first experiencing, appreciating, and being moved by the sunset, one would fail in the experience: the pleasure is a dependent function of the prior experience of beauty. Nor is the experience of beauty itself a mere means to pleasure since, if anything, the beauty "demands" acknowledgment and appreciation on its own terms, before it is productive of pleasure. If anything breaks through our encrusted subjectivity and mere pleasure lust, it is the experience of beauty. A careful phenomenological analysis of experiences of pleasure, including lived body pleasure, demonstrates that many and perhaps most pleasures not only *are not* but *cannot* be experienced without a prior emotional experience of higher values and their appreciation (Scheler, 1973). Hence, the idea that pleasure necessarily functions as a goal seems phenomenologically unfounded, since such pleasures cannot be attained through being a goal but only secondarily through a prior emotional reaction. We note that, once again, lurking in the background of adaptation questions are further questions concerning the nature and hierarchy of values, though again the hierarchy is misapplied in this case.

Freud also assumes a concept of adaptation in his many investigations into sexuality (Rapaport and Gill, 1959). For example, in the first of the *Three Essays on the Theory of Sexuality* (Freud, 1962), Freud discusses sexual aberrations in a manner which suggests that the aberrations are born of maladaptations regarding the expressions of sexuality, including various fixations. This conception of "aberration," one which virtually means the same thing as "maladaptation," assumes not only that adaptation is essential to human development but that there is a psychologically normative sense of adaptation, on the basis of which one's attempt at adaptation can be understood as maladaptive or an aberration. As with any normative concept, there is once again a conception of value at stake in this conception of maladaptation or aberration, just as there are in concepts such as healthy or ill, flourishing or languishing, being vitalized or being "stuck," and other concepts associated with psychic life or health. Indeed, even if contemporary conceptions of what counts as psychologically healthy or ill or what counts as adapted or maladapted might be different from what they are in Freud and in Freud's time, there is always a conception of value behind the notions of adaptation and maladaptation/aberration. In practice, in fact, Freud's classical stages of oral, anal, etc., are understood as progressive levels of adaptation, more or less successfully achieved and measured by such value concepts. Still, as suggested earlier, the working conception of adaptation in this paper is not itself worked through but is assumed: it is taken for granted that life in its progressive and developmental stages consists in challenges to adaptation which a person attains more or less successfully. Furthermore, the successful attainment of adaptation is measured by the possession of certain traits deemed valuable for persons in their maturational process.

A more explicit (rather than assumed) conception of adaptation occurs in Freud's 1924 paper, "The Loss of Reality in Neurosis and Psychosis" (Freud, 1924). One of the most relevant points in this paper is Freud's differentiation of *alloplastic* from *autoplastic* alteration, the former referring to adapting by changing one's environment, the latter adapting by means of changing one's inner life (Hartmann, 1958). This distinction itself has a good deal of merit in that it articulates the two central terms of adaptation: the psyche (or, simply, the person) and the environment in which and, to some extent, toward which one is adapting. The distinction further delineates something about the person's agency, in that it emphasizes that human beings can adapt to their environment but can also in principle change the environment to which they are adapting, or both.

Besides the value of this distinction for Freud's purposes in the paper, we can see there is potential clinical relevance here. After all, often our patients feel stuck, hopeless, or helpless when they also feel powerless to change their environment, including at times needing to walk away from their environment. Often psychological health in a patient hinges on focusing on either the alloplastic or autoplastic side of this distinction, depending on the specifics of the case. While this distinction is useful clinically, it appears too abstract and too metapsychological in the form in which Freud gives it here to be directly relevant to clinical experience. Yet it does highlight one of the general points in this section, namely, that adaptation is present throughout Freud's work, but often in an implicit form or at such a level of generality as to be a helpful metapsychological concept, but not necessarily to contribute much to clinical practice.

Now one could draw the conclusion from this lack of direct analysis that adaptation is not as important an element of classical psychoanalysis as has been suggested throughout this text. In contrast, we would suggest that its importance is seen in the extent to which it is taken for granted. We saw in the previous chapter that the dynamism in the psyche toward adaptation is essential and defining of the psyche and, further, that that was the assumption of the early psychoanalysts, whose work hinged on various philosophies of life characteristic of the nineteenth century. The lack of direct analysis of adaptation in clinical practice in early psychoanalysis is due to the assumption that adaptation is simply and essentially what the psyche does and that one needs no more than to understand what the psyche is to understand its movements and processes as forms of successful or unsuccessful adaptation.

Still, even from this brief discussion of Freud, we can see a few important points that will continue to occupy us for the rest of our study of adaptation. First of all, we have seen that a thorough discussion of adaptation will have at least to make reference to issues associated with value, something which is admittedly not a strong point in the depth psychological tradition. Neither the early psychoanalysts nor the post-existential depth psychologists appear to have a fine-tuned enough notion of value to analyze adaptation. The issue of value from both philosophical and psychological points of view is difficult, and any treatment in this study will have to be cursory and schematic. Yet it will have to be dealt with in some measure, as already our discussions of Freud have suggested. Further, we have seen that such questions of adaptation and value seem necessary not only to Freud's view of development, but to any version of developmental psychology based on stages of development. As a rule, any concept of human development is going to hinge on what counts as successful or unsuccessful adaptation, which in turn assumes some values according to which one measures that success. Finally, we have seen that Freud recognizes the issue of adaptation from both an internal and an external side (i.e., from the standpoint of the inner dynamism toward adaptation and from the standpoint of the environment in which and toward which one adapts). Freud also recognizes a level of agency we have, not only with respect to our inner drive but also over the environment, including some level or capacity to alter the environment for the sake of adaptive success.

Adaptation in Ego Psychology: Heinz Hartmann

In 1937, Heinz Hartmann published an essay entitled "Ego Psychology and the Problem of Adaptation," which appeared largely unchanged and translated into English as the first of a monograph series of the *Journal of the American Psychoanalytic Association* in 1958. The fact that this essay was the "kick-off" essay of a major book series highlights the perception of its quality as an essay. Hartmann begins by underlining the new gains in psychoanalysis through the advent of ego psychology and by attempting to link the work of contemporary psychoanalysis with the work of other yet overlapping disciplines, such as sociology and education. Early on in the book, Hartmann notes that general metapsychological views of psychoanalysis have not fundamentally changed (in his time) but, thanks to recent developments in ego psychology, there is a need to add yet another theoretical and clinical point of view on the psyche and psychic functions, namely, the adaptive point of view. Indeed, Hartmann goes so far as to say that, "adaptation—though we [psychoanalysts and psychoanalytic theorists] do not discuss its implications frequently or thoroughly—is a central concept of psychoanalysis, because many of our problems, when pursued far enough, converge on it" (Hartmann, 1958: p. 22). Perhaps no work before Robert Langs' many texts highlighted the importance of adaptation for Freudian psychoanalytic theory and practice as this work of Hartmann. Despite its importance for our theme, it should be noted that Hartmann's work is largely and consciously metapsychological, whereas the focus in this study is clinical practice. It will be advantageous, therefore, to highlight only those points that appear relevant to our discussions in the ensuing chapters.

Hartmann's opening chapter differentiates between adaptations which entail conflict and those which do not, the latter of which he terms the "conflict-free ego sphere," a sector of psychic life associated with the ego which, nonetheless, as a rule does not cause the kind of conflicts psychoanalysis as a practice generally aims to alleviate. Developmental areas, such as motor skills, are chief constituents of this sphere, by way of example. Hartmann goes on to talk about adaptation in areas where conflict can arise, conceiving adaptation as "reality mastering" (Hartmann, 1958: p. 22) (i.e., the capacity to tolerate conflicts while experiencing life positively).

As Hartmann puts it, "we call a man well adapted if his productivity, his ability to enjoy life, and mental equilibrium are undisturbed" (Hartmann, 1958: p. 23), essentially a definition in terms of work, love, and general psychological health and balance. Hartmann recognizes an important verbal distinction differentiating static and dynamic conceptions of adaptation: he distinguishes between the *state of adaptedness* and the *process of adaptation*. It is one thing to say that someone "is adapted" and another to say that he or she "is adapting" to a situation; the latter, for example, admits of degrees, whereas the former does not. Similarly, adaptation as a process is always "future oriented," something we would not say of adaptedness as a state. This distinction will have at least some relevance in the following as we see that Jung treats adaptation as a process whereas, in contrast, Langs' conception has more to do with the state of adaptedness.

Hartmann's articulation of adaptation parallels our articulation in the previous chapter, in that it suggests a fundamental psychic dynamism prior to and undergirding functional developments of all kinds. Hartmann writes:

> We will clarify matters if we assume that adaptation (speaking now mainly about man) is guaranteed, in both its grosser and finer aspects, on the one hand by man's primary equipment and the maturation of his apparatuses, and on the other hand by those ego-regulated actions which (using this equipment) counteract the disturbances in, and actively improve the person's relationship to, the environment. Man's existing relation to the environment codetermines which of the reactions he is capable of will be used in this process, and also which of the reactions used will predominate. The potentialities and the factual limitations of adaptive processes are already implied here. (Hartmann, 1958: p. 25)

This passage suggests that adaptation is so basic to the movements of the psyche that we can assume not only an adaptive impulse undergirding all psychic life but also that environmental factors codetermine functional actions and reactions (i.e., the possible range of functional activity). In the final chapter, we will discuss the importance of this issue briefly, in terms of potentially useful clinical notions of "fate" versus "destiny."

Hartmann makes much of Freud's distinction between autoplastic and alloplastic change (e.g., Hartmann, 1958: p. 26) (i.e., interior, psychic change versus change to the environment to which one is adapting) in part because the range and extent of human abilities to alter the world alloplastically is "one of the outstanding tasks of human development" (Hartmann, 1958: p. 26)—though Hartmann also notes that not every case of alloplastic alteration is positively adaptive. Though Hartmann only mentions this latter point in passing, it appears to this reader more important than he realizes, if for no other reason because it highlights once again a value hierarchy not defined exclusively by adaptation. Evidently, not everything which might count as a "development" or "successful adaptation" is necessarily a good thing, implying a value scale distinct and independent from a purely descriptive process of adaptation. This point is again hinted at when Hartmann claims that which kind of adaptation, autoplastic or alloplastic, is better often derives from "higher ego function," suggesting an unarticulated but higher standard of evaluation than simply the success of an adaptive process, born of instinctual movements in the psyche, per se.

There can be multiple processes of adaptation in any given case, as when one changes one's environment for the sake of adaptation and then adapts to the new environment, a secondary kind of adaptation. There can also be a form of adaptation which is neither strictly speaking autoplastic or alloplastic, namely, the choice of a new environment entirely. As a side note—or perhaps better described as a side swipe—Hartmann says that the preferred means of adaptation can also be "described crudely in typological terms," a point he follows with a reference to Jung's *Psychological Types* (Hartmann, 1958: p. 26). In chapter 4, we will make the case that Jung's typological differentiation is neither crude nor a mere side point to the issue of adaptation.

Hartmann's articulation of adaptation is in terms of "fitting together" (*Zusammenpassung* in German) with one's environment, in such a way that one can master environmental conditions sufficiently, first of all, to survive and flourish and, second, to do so with some measure of psychological equilibrium. Hartmann highlights that the relationship between organism and environment is always at some point disrupted and that all organisms develop modes of adaptation as a way of managing those disruptions. In the case of human beings, some of those disruptions also produce psychological conflict. Though the human psyche is characteristically elastic and wide-ranging in its adaptive potential, it is also extremely complex and thus highly susceptible to psychic and emotional conflict. Hence adaptation aims at establishing new forms of psychological equilibrium in the face of disruptions to the psyche-environment relationship.

Hartmann differentiates four kinds of equilibrium at which human adaptation aims: (1) equilibrium of person and environment; (2) equilibrium among instinctual drives; (3) equilibrium among psychic functions ("mental institutions"), a kind of structural equilibrium; and (4) equilibrium between the ego's own "synthetic function"—the ego insofar as it is a *force* of equilibrium—and the rest of the ego. While these specific theses, associated as they are with classical ego psychology, are not *a propos* enough to Langs and Jung to merit detailed consideration here, it is key that we recognize the number of potential valences and variables toward which the adaptive process is aimed. The "state of adaptedness," as Hartmann describes it, suggests a complex balancing of a number of different aspects of the ego and of the psyche in general with respect to both inner and outer aspects of life, a point which incidentally parallels Jung more than Langs. Furthermore, though Hartmann's analysis of equilibrium goes a good way toward understanding the various factors involved in adaptive processes, he strangely leaves out the problem of how the psyche and thus psychic equilibrium is not simply an internal and individual phenomenon but also a *social* phenomenon. The psyche is a sensorium not only for individual experiences but also for social (so-called collective) influences and influencing, not to mention social pathology; indeed, the primary adaptive issues we have appear to revolve around other persons and groups, suggesting a still different axis of equilibrium, or at least a very specific application of point (1), which concerns how we hold our own psychological equilibrium in the face of often pathological social systems. We will return to this point, though only briefly, in chapter 5.

Though the immediate goal of adaptation, according to Hartmann, is the "fitting together" of person/psyche and environment, an image borrowed from biological theory, the complexity of human adaptation also shows that the latter is not reducible to biological adaptation: human evolution in part consists in the internalization of processes that were originally external, making what was a purely biological process into a psychological one.

> Here—as so often in biology—on a higher level the same tasks are solved by different means. In phylogenesis, evolution leads to an increased independence of the organism from its environment, so that reactions which originally occurred in relation to the external world are increasingly displaced into the interior of the organism. The development of thinking, of the superego, of the mastery of internal danger before it becomes external, and so forth, are examples of this process of internalization. Thus fitting together (in the psychological realm, the synthetic function) gains in significance in the course of evolution. If we encounter—as we do in man—a function which simultaneously regulates both the environmental relationships and the interrelations of the mental institutions, we will have to place it above adaptation in the biological hierarchy: we will place it above adaptive activity regulated by the external world, that is, above adaptation in the narrower sense but not above adaptation in the broader sense, because the latter already implies a "survival value" determined both by the environmental relationships and the interrelations of mental institutions. (Hartmann, 1958: p. 42–43)

This higher form of adaptation has other implications, according to Hartmann, among others that the "reality principle," under a certain general reading of it, is not merely subordinated to the pleasure principle, but actually has a kind of precedence over the latter. In this way, Hartmann amplifies Freud's notion of the reality principle in a way parallel to our own previous discussions, by suggesting the reality principle has a relatively autonomous value independent of the pleasure principle. Hartmann quotes Freud's *Beyond the Pleasure Principle* to sum up his point, "Both higher development and involution might well be the consequences of adaptation to the pressure of external forces; and in both cases the part played by instincts might be limited to the retention (in the form of an internal source of pleasure) of an obligatory modification" (Hartmann, 1958: p. 45).

Hartmann's essay is a seminal contribution to the theory of adaptation and how it might impact analytic modes of therapy. Hartmann also highlights a situation in his own time that has perhaps not fundamentally changed, namely, that adaptation is implicitly recognized to be a central notion to all psychoanalytic treatment but is taken so much for granted that it is not much examined itself. At the same time, the essay as a whole has less immediate relevance than its title might suggest, because it too, like Freud's essays, is a metapsychological treatise rather than a clinical one. Nonetheless, a number of points Hartmann develops help us focus on the nature of adaptation and set some of the background of how we should understand it in its clinical setting.

For one, Hartmann appears to be on the same page as the analysis in chapter 1, portraying adaptation as perhaps the central dynamism in the psyche, one which underlies psychic functioning in general, and which requires a distinctive point of view on both psychological and metapsychological levels. Hartmann admits that generally psychoanalysis up to his time has not occupied itself with the problem of adaptation, but he also underlines its importance, even considering this recognition one of the hallmark achievements of ego psychology. Hartmann goes so far as to suggest that the basic problems of psychoanalysis all "converge on" the issue of adaptation (Hartmann, 1958: p. 22). Hartmann thus treats adaptation and adaptive issues as a more central issue to psychoanalysis and psychoanalytic theory than anyone previous, making explicit in psychoanalytic theory what has perhaps too often been left implicit.

Second, Hartmann adds to our understanding a sense for the goal of adaptation, namely, what he terms "equilibrium." As Hartmann suggests, this equilibrium is perhaps more an ongoing ideal than an actual achievement and thus it might be that relative equilibrium is all that can be hoped for in practice, in part because life is inherently dynamic and what counts as equilibrium at one point might not count as equilibrium at the next. However, this insight is also important because it gives us a way of analyzing what was imaged in chapter 1 as vital "flow" (i.e., the sense of psychic vitality that accompanies psychological health). This experience of life flowing through us with sufficient energy and robustness that we do not feel "stuck" is a basic factor in psychological life and in many ways a goal of psychotherapy. Hartmann's analysis in terms of various equilibriums gives us a clue to the conditions under which that experience of flow occurs, namely, it occurs when the psyche is functioning with a system of relatively balanced forces within and with a sufficient sense of satisfaction, agency, and mastery without. Clinical problems, as we shall see, are frequently about adaptive challenges to finding such equilibrium, with the goal of experiencing the "flow" that comes only from an equilibrium or from what we shall call a "balance of consciousness" down the line. We will see that Jung offers a similar conception of the goal of adaptation.

Finally, we note here that Hartmann, like Freud, both stated and yet left largely implicit the complex problem of value experiences that in part sets the context of adaptive problems. Hartmann noted that there is another value standard than that of pure adaptive success by which we judge the adaptive achievements. Referring back to the example in the previous chapter: successful adaptation to a pathological system is hardly itself an adaptation positive to the person, since on those conditions, that person will almost certainly share in the systemic pathology. We therefore will have to develop (at least) two different points of view of the value of adaptation—the value of more or less successful adaptation per se and a more global value point of view that asks to what extent such adaptation is conducive to psychological equilibrium and, above all, to a sense of wholeness and individuation.

Conclusion

For the present, we will set aside the specifics of Carl Jung's ideas on adaptation since they are treated as an independent chapter by themselves. Yet it is worthwhile to note that Jung's primary contributions to the issue of adaptation are published after most of those of Freud and predate those of Hartmann and thus could appropriately be a part of this chapter on the older analytic tradition. Further, it is clear that Jung's approach to adaptation was known even in the Freudian world, in that Hartmann at least begrudgingly admits that Jung has something of some significance to say on the issue of adaptation, while simultaneously considering such a treatment "crude." Hence it is clear that Jung's ideas were at least a part of these older discussions. It might be added that, to Hartmann's credit, there is really no denying that Jung's work on the psychological types is often utilized crudely and perhaps invites such usage (in part because of Jung's own inadequate attempts to apply the theory[2]), as when people treat Jung's distinctions among the types as categorial

---

2. Consider, for example, Jung's often strained attempts to reduce differences, say, between thinkers (e.g., Freud and Adler) or between cultures (e.g., "East" and "West"), exclusively to introversion and extraversion. These are good examples of how a groundbreaking thinker may still not be entirely sure of the exact nature and value of his own insights.

descriptions of more or less fixed personalities or personality traits rather than as much subtler attempts to describe adaptive tendencies and functional ranges. However, there is little value in denying the worth of a theory on the grounds that it is sometimes applied crudely, whether we are speaking of Jung or of anyone else. After all, no student of Freud like Hartmann is unfamiliar with similarly crude uses of Freudian psychoanalytic theory both by Freudians and at times by Freud himself.

Hartmann's contribution to the theory of adaptation influenced classical psychoanalytic practice to the point that major figures writing after Hartmann agreed that the "adaptive point of view" had to be added to other classical Freudian viewpoints on clinical theory and practice, such as topographical, structural, economic, etc. (Rapaport and Gill, 1959; Greenson, 1967). It is probably in the wake of these developments, at least in North American psychoanalysis, that questions concerning how adaptation practically and concretely impacts clinical practice came to the fore. Merton Gill was in fact one of the leading figures in this "movement" (if that is the right word), though he was also critical of a number of elements of Langs' teaching (Gill, 1984). But perhaps the most famous and the most prolific was Langs himself, to whom we shall turn in a moment.

One irony concerning the effects of Hartmann's work is that, though Langs clearly works in the wake of that tradition, he does not seem to draw much of anything directly or literally from Heinz Hartmann. Indeed, I brought Hartmann up to Langs in an email once, shortly before Langs' death, asking if he was aware of Hartmann's treatise on adaptation (which I knew he must be), because I had never noticed a reference to Hartmann in Langs' work. Langs' response was cursory and perhaps dismissive, suggesting that, yes, he of course knew of Hartmann's treatise, but didn't feel it had much to say about what Langs was interested in. On one level, that was an understandable reaction from Langs: generally, Langs' work is very clinically oriented and Hartmann's treatise is not, aiming at general, metapsychological propositions rather than concrete clinical and technical details.

However, at another level, it is somewhat surprising that Langs did not refer to Hartmann virtually at all or allow much by way of influence from Hartmann. For one, Langs always proudly called himself a "classical psychoanalyst," a term which would suggest that Langs saw himself to be very much in the tradition of which Hartmann is a prime representative (though one can reasonably debate the value of the term "classical psychoanalyst" for Langs, as in Gill [1984]). One might wonder if the lack of impact on his work by someone like Hartmann arises from the fact that, in his early career, Langs tended to take the traditional metapsychology and philosophical assumptions of classical analysis for granted and focus very minutely on clinical experiences and interactions, whereas later in his career, Langs would draw the conclusion that he needed a new metapsychology, would drop much of the classical metapsychology and philosophical assumptions of the Freudian tradition, and articulate his own—and do so in great detail.

The later directions of Langs' metapsychology will not occupy us in this study, but it is worth highlighting that Langs may have missed an opportunity. Among Hartmann's strengths in this treatise is a sense for the overall development of the human being through adaptation, whereas Langs' tendency was always to see the value of adaptive problems only in the clinical moment, in the very concrete events within clinical sessions. As we will suggest in the final chapter, Langs undercut some of his own best insights by focusing so minutely on clinical interaction that the longitudinal well-being of his patients did not seem to factor into his clinical studies or his conception of clinical technique. One of Langs' strengths was his ability to isolate and highlight sometimes minute parts of the clinical process, but his correlating weakness, it would seem, was a lack of focus on the overall process of the patient and how that general movement and change impacts the same minutiae of clinical practice. For example, Hartmann's fine-tuned if brief analysis of forms of psychological equilibrium could only really have been studied clinically from the standpoint of long-term development, since we could not expect equilibriums of this sort to be a constant or to occur in a simple clinical moment, but to be the development of longer-term psychological trends going on in the patient. The methodological approach Langs took to his clinical studies all but forbade the kind of clinical view one would have to take to understand a notion like psychological equilibrium. In this respect, we will find that Jung is closer to Hartmann than Langs is.

CHAPTER 3

Robert Langs and Adaptation in Clinical Practice

Introduction

As we have seen, adaptation is a notion clearly present yet usually implicit within the broader psychoanalytic tradition. The advent of ego psychology brought with it a focus on the singular importance of adaptation, though much of that focus was metapsychological in nature, doing little to elucidate the clinical consequences of adaptation. The psychoanalyst who has done perhaps the most to work out the clinical significance of adaptation was not an ego psychologist per se, but proudly self-identified as a "classically-trained psychoanalyst," Robert Langs. We begin with a few brief and relevant biographical points.

Langs trained at one of the premier psychoanalytic training centers in his time, the Downstate Medical Center, from 1959 to 1968. Among his teachers was the internationally known analyst and author Jacob Arlow, whose work emphasized the importance of subliminal (unconscious) perception, a notion of central importance to all of Langs' work. Langs' first book, his two-volume set *The Technique of Psychoanalytic Psychotherapy*, illustrates well both the assumptions of (what Langs termed) "classical psychoanalysis" and its clinical practices at the time, as well as Langs' own original articulation of the same. Yet even in this text, Langs deviates from that tradition he proudly identified with (e.g., by seeing psychoanalysis and psychoanalytic psychotherapy as functionally the same regarding technique). For the first twenty or so years of his writing career (early 1970s to mid-1990s), Langs believed his work was *modifying* classical psychoanalysis, mostly by emphasis, and did not represent a new and unique form of psychoanalysis distinct from classical psychoanalysis. In fact, many of the basic tenets of classical psychoanalysis permeate Langs' work, both early and late, even as Langs attempts to underline elements of the tradition that he thinks are more basic and foundational than standard classical psychoanalytic theory and practice took them to be. Though Langs deviates from classical psychoanalytic theory in certain respects—early on, for example, in his insistence on the primacy of adaptive issues and, later, in his rooting of psychic conflict in trauma and death anxiety—Langs nonetheless remains solidly within the classical psychoanalytic tradition *clinically speaking*, including in his basic conception of the unconscious as something emerging implicitly in the manifest clinical content of sessions.

More substantial changes in Langs' thought emerge through the 1990s and beyond. At this later point, Langs' use of classical psychoanalytic theoretical concepts, such as drive theory, ego, object-relations, and so forth, diminishes, in favor of his own newly developing terminology predicated on his "adaptive paradigm" and its emphasis on trauma and death anxiety. In the last phase of his work, Langs not only rejects Freud's structural trichotomy of ego-superego-id but interprets the latter theory as a formation arising from Freud's defense against his own death anxiety—one of the subjects of Langs' last published book (Langs, 2010).

Given these differences in Langs' long career, it might seem *a propos* to treat Langs' work in different phases. However, a careful reading of Langs' work throughout the more than forty years of his publications suggests that his clinical practice and theory changed a good deal less than the broader psychoanalytic and theoretical framework in which the clinical theory was embedded. Though a treatment of Langs' work in its totality could indeed only be done adequately in phases, focusing on his clinical theory alone permits us to treat it largely as a unit. This is so because the changes in Langs' clinical theory are mostly reinterpretations of the same practices and the same clinical data, rather than fundamental changes in the practices and data themselves. For example, Langs' early treatments of the unconscious imply that the unconscious is not only a receptacle of repressed contents but also communicates essential clinical insight to the therapist. In his later work, he articulates distinct conceptualizations and terminology, distinguishing the "unconscious" in the usual psychoanalytic sense from what he calls the "deep unconscious," the first correlating to the Freudian unconscious, the latter to the "wisdom system" (Langs' term) from which one gains clinical insight about a specific treatment in therapy—a concept, incidentally, not entirely different from Jung's notion of the Self. Though the latter terminology is new in the late 1990s, it is in practice only a new way of conceptualizing what Langs was already saying in the 1970s, not a substantive change in the actual practice or clinical theory.

Consequently, we will treat Langs' adaptive clinical theory as a unit, offering a general outline of the theory and its most salient characteristics, followed by a brief excursus highlighting one way in which Langs' later clinical theory does imply an alteration, yet not so much in concrete practice as in what one is listening for in clinical material. We will also illustrate Langs' method with an extended piece of a clinical case.

Original Development of Adaptation and the "Adaptive Context"

Langs wrote a substantial retrospective piece a mere ten years into his analytic career, as the introduction to a volume collecting his previously published papers. The retrospective was entitled, like the volume itself, "Technique in Transition" (Langs, 1978a), and it reconsiders the changing dynamics of his thought (Langs, 1978a: p. 5). Langs refers to two chapters of the volume as "early papers," though published only six and five years previously, respectively, suggesting his perception of being in an entirely new phase in his work and his sense of significant alterations in his thinking at the time this essay was written. Those two early essays represent the psychoanalytic orthodoxy of the time, according to Langs, whereas the rest of the volume consists of papers indicative of "profound changes" in his work and thus significant deviations from classical psychoanalysis and technique. Speaking of the entire volume, Langs writes that these papers

> were written over the relatively brief span of seven years, and yet contain, I believe, a series of interrelated transitions in conception and technique with far-reaching consequences for both the patient and the therapist or analyst. (Langs, 1978a: p. 3)

What changed so drastically between the early 1970s Langs and the current Langs of 1978? It was the recognition of the significance of adaptation for all analytically oriented clinical work. Langs underwent a series of theoretical transitions, motivated by the insight that clinical material and psychic conflict can best be understood in terms of adaptation (i.e., the attempt on the part of the psyche to react and respond to environmental situations which require significant change on the patient's part, emotionally, cognitively, and/or behaviorally). Hence, psychic conflict for Langs is always in part a function of an unsuccessful attempt to adapt.

Adaptation was so important a concept for Langs that he believed all clinical material required organization in its terms, that one can only understand clinical material, and especially the unconscious communications embedded in it, by relating such material to adaptive contexts. Langs' empirical foundation for his claims is not only his own clinical work but even more his observations of clinical material given by supervisees. By way of example, Langs mentions that he went through more than three hundred hours of recorded clinical sessions for the second paper of the anthology (Langs, 1978a: p. 10) and found that, by looking for the primary "adaptive context" or, as he later calls it, the "trigger," he could make sense of the various materials which were present, something he could not do without considering the adaptive context. Writing about the development of his concept of adaptation, Langs writes:

> In the dream paper [one of the "early papers" mentioned earlier], I had found that the day residue was often the crucial organizer through which the

unconscious meaning took shape and could be recognized. In evaluating other types of communication—conscious fantasies, descriptions of recent events, that patient's behaviors, etc.—I found that, globally, I could identify a series of meaningful surface indicators of problems, conflicts, and resistances quite readily; on the other hand, the material appeared confused and difficult to decipher for specific unconscious fantasies and memories. The confusion was resolved, however, when I extended the day residue concept to a search for reality precipitants in every sequence of material. These precipitants turned out to be major adaptive tasks confronting the patient; it was soon evident that some of these tasks evoked relatively realistic and nonpathological responses, while others set off a sequence of unconscious fantasies and memories, almost all of which were essentially related to the patient's pathology and inner anxieties and conflicts. (Langs, 1978a: p. 10)

The recognition that adaptation is the chief organizer of clinical material became, according to Langs, "undoubtedly the single most important concept I have developed" (Langs, 1978a: p. 11).

Langs did not change his evaluation of the importance of adaptation for understanding clinical material and process throughout the rest of his forty-some-year career. Nearer to the end of his career, Langs refers to his approach as the "adaptive paradigm" and, as time goes on, he distinguishes it sharply from standard psychoanalytic approaches. In some later papers, he will differentiate what he calls "weak adaptive" approaches (e.g., classical psychoanalysis and, implicitly, Jungian analysis) from his own "strong adaptive" approach, where adaptive issues are neither left implicit nor treated as one principle among many but are treated as the sole and central organizer of clinical material and psychic life (Langs, 2005). Throughout the at times labyrinthine ways of Langs' changing conceptions through the years, the primacy of adaptation for clinical practice does not waver, even if he develops other important concepts and theoretical notions throughout his decades of clinical research.

The previous-quoted passage in Langs' text highlights ideas and themes Langs utilizes throughout his career, some which are worth underlining. First, Langs assumes an implicit opposition between "reality precipitants" or, if you will, just "reality," and what we might term "irreal" psychic phenomena, such as unconscious fantasy, memories, and so forth. Langs' model here, evidently derived from the hard sciences of the time, tended to be strongly materialistic, treating "reality" as something coextensive with material factors. Langs' earliest publications were not in clinical theory but in empirical psychiatric research (investigations concerning patients' use of LSD) and he never seems to have lost a somewhat materialistic, scientific (at times even "scientistic") bent. Evidently in the spirit of the psychiatric science of the time, Langs adheres to a sharp opposition between the *reality* of the external material world and the *irreality* of the fantasy life of the internal world, an opposition he hangs on to for his entire scholarly life.

The significance of this opposition should not be lost on us because most of the criticisms Langs raises against classical psychoanalysis revolve around the idea that classical psychoanalysis does not sufficiently recognize the importance of reality in its understanding of psychic life. When Langs offers examples of this criticism, they are typically cases of interpretations formulated in purely intrapsychic terms, rather like the example we gave in the opening chapter where my peer proposed the image of a bull and a few associations and treated them as the clinical material of the presentation. Langs would say that, without at least a hypothesized adaptive context or trigger, there is no way to grasp the inherent meaning of the psychic event in question, in part because the material is therefore not associated with reality.[1]

While Langs' conception might at times be useful, it also runs some risks of its own. For one, it becomes clear that Langs thinks of psychodynamics as a purely internal, intrapsychic study, whereas adaptation is the study of what relates the psyche to the external, real world. Langs is evidently not alone in this understanding of psychodynamics, as we can see for example in standard criticisms relational psychoanalysts make against Freud, as if the latter works out the dynamics of the psyche while enclosed, as it were, in a Cartesian mental prison, cut off from relationship and the outer world (Mills, 2010). Whatever the merit of those criticisms by relational psychoanalysts, what we can certainly say is that some significant body of American psychoanalysts read psychodynamics as if it is a wholly internal study and, in Langs' case, the "way out" of that internal trap is by the study of adaptation, which relates the psyche to the external and real world.[2]

However, while such an approach may solve one set of problems it raises another set, namely, how are these two purportedly diverse studies—psychodynamics and adaptation—connected to each other? This author sees little phenomenological basis for thinking the internal and external worlds are quite so separable as Langs' conception suggests; quite the contrary, inner and outer worlds are often intertwined in meaningful unities in a way that can neither justify the idea that psychodynamics is purely internal or that adaptation is a purely external process. We will discuss this in more detail in chapter 4.[3]

A further issue this passage from Langs raises is the question of whether reality is coextensive with material reality; if so, then there is no place for

---

1. Kugler and Hillman (1985) make a similar point in criticism of Goodheart's assimilation of Langs, though in a more general way, that is, by pointing out that there are implicit and differentiated ontologies (conceptions of reality) assumed at the outer and inner levels. In my terminology, their point is that this it is not an issue of real versus irreal but what form of reality is at stake.

2. This is not to say that there no signs of an internal sort of adaptation in Langs as, for example, his discussion of the "structure of emotional disturbance" suggests (Langs, 1982). Yet even then, Langs' never quite convinces this reader that he considers internal adaptation an important or ultimate source of emotional disturbance. In the end, adaptive contexts are external because they are real, rather than irreal.

3. Kugler and Hillman (1985) have given a far more thorough critique of Goodheart and Langs on ontological grounds than the hints I am giving here.

non-material reality, such as the psyche. As was argued in chapter 1, adaptation is possible because it is predicated of a *real* psyche: the relationship between the (real) adapting psyche and the (real) environment to which it adapts. Thus both successful and unsuccessful adaptation hinge not only on the outer, "external" reality to which one adapts but on the content of one's "inner" reality, including one's psychic history, dominant complexes, psychic structure, and other related factors—none of which are themselves irreal fantasies and all of which must be understood as real characteristics of a very real psyche. Though these real, inner factors certainly do *produce* conscious fantasies, unconscious phantasies, dreams, and the like, some of which could aptly be described as "irreal," it does not follow that the psyche producing them does not have a type of reality of its own, even if that reality is not of the material variety. Just as little as one could validly infer from the fact that the character Hamlet is not real that therefore the mind of Shakespeare was not real, could one infer from the irreal character of fantasy that the psyche producing it is not itself real. Quite the contrary, such fantasy products also indicate important structural features about the nature, status, and active complexes of the psyche. The failure here to acknowledge what Jung called "the reality of the psyche" leads Langs, I will suggest, to too one-sided an approach to adaptation, something which the contrast of his position to that of Jung will highlight.

This tendency on Langs' part also undermines his understanding of the nature of psychic conflict. At times, for example, the genuine adaptive issue may have very little to do with the externals per se but have a lot to do with what relating to those externals provokes in one's internal life. For example, I may be filled with anxiety because I have actual tax problems and I am not sure how to adapt to them. That is a definite adaptive issue which includes the reality of taxes. But I may not have any actual tax issues, yet still find that even thinking about doing my taxes provokes unconscious negative father phantasies which arise in general with my experiences of authority, such as that of the Internal Revenue Service. It is both important, in such a case, to recognize that the external adaptive context co-defines and occasions the problem by provoking the complexes in specific ways but equally important to see that the dominant element producing the psychic conflict may not be the external occasion or "reality precipitant," but the internal reality to which this external reality correlates, the father complex. In this case, we can say that the psyche is "adapted" when it can manage through its own inner resources to do the taxes and live with the consequences, while not acting primarily and unconsciously from the activated father complex. That it is tax time when this complex is provoked is, in this second case, more an occasion than an adaptive cause of the psychological distress. Points of this kind will occupy us down the road, as we suggest that inner and outer sides of adaptive situations are not two separable factors but meaningful psychological unities which, nonetheless, can entail a certain priority on one side or the other of the given adaptive context.

Whatever the potential weaknesses, these points from Langs' early work give us not only a sense of how Langs developed his idea of the primacy of adaptation, but also why he did so. Langs found that, once the issue of adaptation was raised, clinical material, especially the unconscious phantasies and meanings, became intelligible; without raising the issue of the adaptive context and the relationship between the inner conflicts and their outer motivating factors, no such intelligibility was to be found. For this reason, it is difficult to overrate how important Langs experienced and thought adaptive issues to be. In practice, Langs believed, all approaches to unconscious material that leave out the question of the adaptive context are equivalent to having no key for understanding the material in any meaningful sense: adaptive contexts amount to the Rosetta Stone of the unconscious, for Langs, and act in many respects as the criterion of valid interpretive interventions. It is for this reason more than others, perhaps, that Langs polemically calls all therapy which does not begin with adaptation as its basic principle "lie therapy," a therapy founded on the false premise that something other than adaptive problems primarily illuminates psychic conflict and thus potentially produces psychic healing.[4]

Central Ideas Derived from Langs' Understanding of Adaptation

Once Langs came to recognize the importance of adaptation to external reality for understanding unconscious material, it modified how he understood many of the basic tenets and techniques of psychoanalytic psychotherapy. The following elements of Langs' clinical theory develop on the basis of his insight into the clinical primacy of adaptive issues and constitute some of the consistent and defining features in Langs' work. Naturally, these can only be treated schematically in a text of this length.

Rearticulating the Analytic Relationship

Among the developments in Langs' thinking is his own adaptation of the Barangers' (1966) ideas on the therapeutic interaction as a *field*. In general, Langs' earliest works assume the traditional analytic and psychiatric approach, which focuses exclusively on the patient and which also tends to underrate the contributions of the analyst to the analytic experience, such as we discussed in the chapter 1. In this respect, Langs, as it were, catches up to Jung who, already in his clinical papers from the 1930s, recognizes the interactive character of clinical experience, a notion Jung further develops in greatest detail in his *Psychology of the Transference*. The Barangers' paper, entitled "Insight in the Analytic Situation," was

---

4. Langs borrows this language of "truth and lie therapy" from Bion (1970) though evidently using it in a somewhat different sense. See also Grotstein (1984).

a breakthrough in psychoanalytic literature because it uses a dyadic rather than monadic understanding of the clinical situation. This paper helps Langs to formulate what he terms the "bi-personal field," a notion which suggests that clinical experience was the work of two, mutually adapting persons (Langs, 1976; Grotstein, 1984).

Langs' developing notion of the role of both "reality precipitants" and adaptation in understanding the therapeutic relationship was further reinforced and expanded by his reading of the work of Harold Searles (Langs and Searles, 1980). Searles' research suggests that unconscious interaction occurs all the time in therapy and analysis, a point Searles develops with regard, for example, to how a patient tries unconsciously to make the therapist into the therapist the patient needs. Hence, if one admits on principle that analysis is not simply about intrapsychic experiences on the part of the patient but is also about "external reality" and how one responds and adapts to it, it is an unavoidable conclusion that the therapeutic relationship *itself* is a significant reality to which one must adapt. In the end, the therapist is neither a neutral observer nor simply an interpreter of the patient's intrapsychic experiences. Rather the therapist and their interventions are motivating factors in the patient's psychic life, factors which evoke adaptive reactions on the part of the patient, just as the therapist is also simultaneously reacting and adapting to the patient in turn (Gill, 1984). Langs came to believe that the therapist as a rule looms larger in the patient's psychic life than any other figure, at least during the period of treatment. This being the case, the therapeutic situation must be understood interactively, an approach which broke with the classical psychoanalytic view of the time, though it gained in popularity in the following decades thanks in part to Searles' growing fame and to movements within the psychoanalytic tradition, such as relational psychoanalysis and allied approaches.

While Langs' development of the interactive dimension of psychotherapy is certainly an advance in many respects, the discussions up to this point already highlight some of its deficits. For one, it appears questionable whether this mutual adaptation should be understood in strictly and exclusively external terms, especially if adaptation is not only about external reality but also internal resources for adaptation, a point which will be emphasized when we look at Jung's theory of adaptation. Furthermore, though mutual adaptation might be an apt description of the interaction, Langs' treatment still gives the impression that the psychological life of each member of the clinical dyad is simply enclosed "within," with only the adaptive process occurring without. If, in contrast, psychic life is always projecting itself into the world and into the immediate psychological environment, as suggested in chapter 1, Langs does not sufficiently take into account that the adaptive process refers not only to the physical but also to the *psychic* environment in the room—an idea his materialistic tendencies probably would not countenance. This side of Langs is also bound up with another assumption highlighted in chapter 1, namely, that the unconscious is somehow simply "within" the patient and analyst, rather than something which falls between the cracks of a largely Empiricist ontology of discrete material things.

The "Reality" of Therapy Includes the Therapeutic Frame

Langs recognized the importance of the "therapeutic frame" early on in his analytic career. By "frame" Langs refers to all those conditions of therapy which, though not themselves the therapeutic interaction, are intrinsic to making the interaction possible as well as making it secure (Langs, 1979; Langs, 1982; Langs, 2005).[5]

Thus among the reality precipitants for adaptation in therapy are included not only responses of the patient to the therapist but also to the elements of the therapeutic frame, which set an adaptive context in which psychotherapy and analysis can happen. There can easily be a tendency among mental health professionals to think that therapeutic work consists simply and exclusively in the interaction of patient and therapist, when in practice all the conditions that enter into functioning psychotherapy, ranging over cost; manner of fee payment; time constraints; traveling; issues of note-taking; third-party (such as insurance company or employer) knowledge; whether the therapy occurs in a private, agency, or home setting; and many other factors are also psychologically internal to the therapeutic process, because each can and often does carry unconscious meanings for both patient and therapist. Hence, Langs believes that each of these elements of the frame are equal parts of therapeutic reality to which the patient must adapt in order to be engaged in therapy and that they are therefore always potential candidates for unconscious communication and interpretation. As Langs' work develops, he if anything puts more emphasis on the frame because he believes it to be an underrated area of unconscious perception and meaning.

We will have occasion to return to Langs' conception of the frame in the final chapter.[6] At this point, it can at least be pointed out that Langs neither seems to question whether what he terms the "secure frame" could at all change its form through a given therapeutic process or to question whether successful analytic work has, as one of its consequences, that the frame becomes more an internalized than external phenomenon.

---

5. The image of the "frame" appears to derive from Milner (1952).

6. Cwik (2010) analyzes three metaphors for analytic structure (the "frame" being one of them), highlighting the strengths and the shadows of each metaphor. Cwik correctly points out that the frame metaphor can give too rigid a sense of analytic structure, at least in certain cases, which contrasts with the other two metaphors of "holding" and "container." My suspicion is that Langs—who knew the language of "holding"—preferred "frame" in part because it had connotations of material reality and, thus, would sound more like an adaptive trigger, on his model, than, for example, "holding" would.

The Communicative Fields

One area where Langs' clinical research has had a decisive influence on Jungian practice is his theory of communicative fields, this influence being mediated through the outstanding articulation and development of Langs' theory by the Jungian William Goodheart (Goodheart, 1980). Goodheart not only used Langs' ideas in a largely unaltered form, but also related Langs' analysis of communicative fields to Jungian concepts and thought. Langs' development of the nature of therapeutic communication and communicative fields was important enough that he at times opted to call his theory the "communicative approach" rather than the "adaptive approach." In the end, the "adaptive approach" won out, however, because Langs felt that the communicative elements in the therapeutic field are themselves functions of adaptation.[7]

Premising his ideas on the point that therapy occurs in a field between analyst and patient, Langs distinguishes between three kinds of *communicative* fields in therapy and analysis (Langs, 1978; Langs, 1980a; Langs, 1982). These fields are always in some measure co-constituted, because of the adaptive and interactive nature of therapeutic practice. Nonetheless, the fields describe modes of communicative style which can also differ between analyst and patient, as when one of them is communicating in one field and the other in another field. No single patient or session is always in one of the fields, but each moves along the various axes of these three types of communicative fields, sometimes in a way that causes communicative breakdowns due to the patient or analyst communicating in a different mode than the other realizes. Further, though one of these types of communicative field (Type A) is considered the best for analytic work proper, it is also relatively unstable and difficult to retain and thus requires vigilance and tending on the part of the therapist or analyst (Goodheart, 1980). The three basic categories of communication Langs calls (none too descriptively) Types A, B, and C fields; Goodheart later denominates them "secured-symbolizing field" (Type A), "complex-discharging field" (Type B), and "persona-restoring field" (Type C) (Goodheart, 1980).

Langs develops these fields over the space of hundreds of pages of supervision transcripts and then summarizes them in his book *Psychotherapy: A Basic Text* (1982). To put his development in as succinct form as possible, we could differentiate them according to the basic principle of how one—either analyst or patient—*relates to his or her own emotional energy*. For example, one who inhibits relationship to his or her own emotionally charged psyche produces a Type C or persona-restoring field because, by virtue of suppression, repression, or other mechanisms and defenses, one is cut off from one's emotional life and therefore cannot produce symbols and images of analytic value. In such a case, one is not

---

7. Langs bases his differentiation of communicative fields in part on Searles' work. Goodheart highlights a number of parallels (1980).

really connected to what Jung calls the "shadow" (i.e., the decisive com-plexed and affectively charged elements and disturbances that remain uncon-scious, just beneath the surface of consciousness) in favor of an inauthentic, persona-rooted (non-)relationship to emotional life. According to Langs, this communicative field is not conducive to analytic work proper (e.g., working with images, symbols, and dreams), in part because this field is designed for "non-communication" (Langs, 1978) and requires, as a rule, non-analytic types of therapy and therapeutic stances.[8]

The person who "acts out" emotional life and conflict in session produces a Type B or complex-discharging field. In this case, the issue is not that one is not connected with one's emotional life, as in the Type C field, but rather that one cannot tolerate the frustration of holding and carrying the energy charge of one's emotional life, venting the charge through acting out or projecting, living out emotional conflict without a sufficiently developed observing ego to stand above it. Langs describes this field as "an action discharge field in which projective identification predominates. In it, either the patient or the analyst makes extensive use of projective identifications designed to rid the psyche of disturbing accretions of inner stimuli, to make use of the other member of the dyad as a container for disrupting projective identifications" (Langs, 1978a). As in the case of the Type C field, here too the communicative field is not con-ducive to standard analytic forms of therapy, according to Langs, but for a different reason: because the energy which could go into the unconscious to produce symbols and images is instead frittered away by being acted out in projection and projective identification.[9]

In contrast, the Type A or secured-symbolizing field is produced when one is both (1) in contact with one's emotional life (in contrast to a Type C field) and (2) rather than acting the emotional charge out, the energy of that charge is contained sufficiently, such that it awakens the image- and symbol-producing power of the unconscious (in contrast to the Type B field). It is in this secured-symbolizing field that one does psychoanalytic work proper, according to Langs.

For Langs, not only the analyst-patient dyad but also the frame needs to be secure enough to make a Type A field possible, since the communi-cative field is itself a product of interactive adaptation and a secured ther-apeutic environment: in this respect, the outer secure frame is in essence representative of an inner secure frame (see chapter 5), which permits the toleration of frustration and a purely psychological use of emotional energy. For example, even if a patient can both contain and be related to their emotional life and concomitant energy charges, the Type A or

---

8. Goodheart notes that Jung's concept of the "regressive restoration of the persona" falls into this type of communicative situation.

9. One could debate whether Langs' critical view of this second form of communicative field is as resistant to analytic work as he suggests. Henry Z'vi Lothane, for example, has developed a dramatological approach to psychoanalysis which could be quite conducive to working with this communicative field (Lothane, 2009; Lothane, 2011).

secured-symbolizing field will not be constituted if the frame is so porous that patient and analyst are having to adapt to inconsistent or anti-therapeutic environmental factors during the analytic work.

In his later work, Langs abandoned the three-fold distinction of communicative field in favor of a two-fold distinction, namely, between narrative and non-narrative forms of communication—though this difference is not necessarily a change in principle, in that Types B and C fields would each constitute non-narrative forms of communication (Langs, 2004).[10] Langs came to believe that what he had previously termed the Type A field could only be communicated narratively (i.e., in the manner of a story) and that any other form of communication was in principle not a Type A field; hence any non-narrative form of communication invariably implied communicative deviations from the ideal type of therapeutic and analytic communication (Langs, 2005). In his later practice, Langs would often have patients simply invent a story in session and then develop the themes of the story through associations, just as one might do with a dream. In this respect, Langs very much deviated from some tenets of classical analysis by demanding of the patient some specific activity (story-making) and yet, in another way, he did so in order to guarantee that another basic tenet of classical analytic therapy was intact, namely, a communicative field which would be symbolic in nature.

At this point, we only note that the communicative field in Langs' work appears to be more or less exclusively a *linguistic* field, a point we will return to in a moment.

Unconscious Communication and Analytic Listening

Langs investigated the issue of unconscious communication in great detail. For Langs, as for Freud and for most Jungians, the dream is, so to speak, the ideal case of unconscious communication. However, as Freud already recognized in his own time, analytic practitioners cannot depend on dreams for all or even most of the unconscious material derived in analysis and therapy, in part because many patients rarely or never bring dreams and in part because, even if there are dreams, not every patient is psychologically in a place where working the dream is feasible or effective. Traditionally, therefore, psychoanalysts have turned to four other sources for unconscious material, the transference, free associations, derivative communication, and the therapist's countertransference.[11]

---

10. Langs noted to me in a personal communication that he didn't see this difference as a change in principle but rather emphasizing the real difference between the Type A field, on the one hand, from the other two types.

11. As is generally known, the positive value of the countertransference only emerged relatively recently in the tradition, decades after the inception of psychoanalysis as a practice (see, e.g., Akhtar, 2012).

As we have noted, Langs spends hundreds of pages analyzing the interactive dyad of patient and therapist and, in the process, gained a good deal of clarity concerning the therapeutic relationship. Among the most important points that Langs emphasizes is that, if we mean by "transference" the pathological elements of a therapeutic relationship, we must understand the transference to be in principle only a part of the therapeutic relationship as a whole: besides transferential or pathological elements, there are also genuine *perceptions* on the part of a patient's unconscious. We can see how this point is essentially a consequence of the assumption that there are real and adaptive dimensions of the analytic relationship. If that latter assumption is true, then not everything in the therapeutic relationship is likely to be "transference" in the pathological sense because the latter is always in some measure illusory; hence some of the therapeutic relationship (except perhaps in extreme psychopathology) is almost certainly accurately perceived, including—at least potentially—perceptions of clinical errors on the part of the therapist. It is therefore incumbent on the therapist or analyst to consider clinical material not only as potentially transferential but also as potentially accurate and to try to discern which it is in any given case (Langs, 1978; Langs, 1982).

The primary medium for unconscious material, for Langs, is derivative communication, something we must learn to listen for and understand through what he will later in his career term *trigger decoding*. Some discussion therefore of both derivative communication and trigger decoding is necessary. "Derivative communication" is an important part of classical psychoanalytic therapy but is not always emphasized among Jungians. The concept of derivative communication is predicated on the Freudian idea that, like dreams, language can have both a latent and manifest content: a manifest level of communication that is largely straightforward and conscious and also a second level of partially disguised communication, which is latent and unconscious. Not every form of verbal communication, according to Langs, can have this two-fold structure; in practice, these communications will only occur within Type A (secured-symbolizing) communicative fields (Langs, 1978; Langs, 1982) and, as he will later say, more or less exclusively in narrative forms of communication (Langs, 2004). Interpreting derivative communication hidden within these narratives is, for Langs, the basic work of the therapist.

Goodheart offers a straightforward example of this sort of communication. A therapist feels that therapy is not going well and brings it up to the patient, who in turn denies there is any problem. Immediately after, the patient tells the story of his business partner and the problems they have communicating with each other. This material is told in the narrative form, as a story, and speaks of a partnership with communicative challenges. Assuming Langs' theory, we can easily hypothesize that, though the manifest content is about the patient's business and business partner, the story is also a disguised communication suggesting ways in which the "business" of therapy is not working, since the theme concerns an interpersonal dyad and communicative malfunctioning—a fairly good description of problematic therapy. According to Langs, therapy is *always* fair game as an adaptive context and always looms largest among possible adaptive contexts. Perhaps this very schematic example is sufficient for the moment to understand derivative communication and how it might be discerned in patient material.

Langs suggests that we "decode" derivative communications by watching for two things (besides the adaptive context): (1) the themes of the narrative and (2) the tone of the narrative (Langs, 2004). Concerning the first, one can begin to discern the derivative communication by extracting the theme from the conscious narrative and asking whether that theme could apply to an adaptive problem in therapy or, secondarily, to an adaptive context in life as a whole. In the example of the previous paragraph, Goodheart presupposes an adaptive context of problems in therapy which in turn illuminates the latent communication, expressed by the theme of a communication-challenged partnership. Because the therapy doesn't seem to be working, the therapist can assume it likely that the latter is a trigger for unconscious communication, not only because of what is happening in the patient's life but also because of a parallel process going on in therapy, one that the patient probably feels too uncomfortable to admit to himself and/or to the analyst or therapist.

The *tone* of the narrative is also key for decoding its meaning. Since the affective tone in the patient's story is negative, one assumes that the unconscious communication is about something that isn't going right, where adaptation is not successful. If, in contrast, the patient tells a story with a positive tone, the unconscious communication would suggest that therapy or something else in the patient's life has "gone right," that adaptation is working.

These two valences of derivative communication—theme and tone— aid the analyst both in understanding the derivative communications and in evaluating therapeutic interventions. Concerning the latter, if an analyst intervenes during a session with, say, an interpretation of the patient's material, the material that follows the interpretation will tend to validate or invalidate it. If, for example, after an interpretation, a patient begins to tell stories of blind or deaf relatives, misunderstandings among people, thick-headed co-workers, or similar themes, one can usually infer that the intervention was incorrect, because the theme suggests miscommunication. Similarly, if the tone of the stories recounted suggest something negative, it is often an indication that the intervention was not correct or was largely incorrect. In contrast, if stories of positive or affirmative relationships, feeling understood, healing, etc., arise, or again, if positive-toned stories arise in the patient's material, chances are that the intervention offered is basically correct. This highlights perhaps the most distinctive element of Langs' work, his way of listening to material and the intervening sequence: listening-intervening-validating (Langs, 1978).[12]

Going back to the earlier point about transferential versus non-transferential elements of the therapeutic relationship, we can see that this approach to derivative communication must play the central role in Langs' work, a role somewhat different from classical psychoanalytic practice. Langs relies on unconscious communications to discover (1) where there are transferential issues, (2) how and when to intervene, and (3) whether the interventions are valid. Though working with derivatives is not new in the psychoanalytic tradition, Langs' evaluation of their importance and the many ways in which he uses them is (Gill, 1984). It is, for example, often assumed by psychoanalytic practitioners that a patient giving more material after an intervention of itself validates the intervention. In contrast, Langs thinks the nature and quality of the further material is what validates or invalidates the intervention (Langs, 2004). A further difference from classical psychoanalysis is that, for Langs, the unconscious cannot simply be a storehouse of repressed memories and feelings nor simply elements of the ego, superego, or id of which one is unaware. Rather, Langs insists that the "unconscious" includes what he will later call a "wisdom system" (Langs, 2004; Langs, 2005), which guides therapeutic practice, something the therapist or analyst recognizes via the listening-intervening-validating sequence. In this respect, in fact, Langs was closer to Jung than he recognized, granting a positive, guiding role to unconscious processes, paralleling Jung's notion of the Self. In his final book, *Freud on a Precipice*, Langs articulates some of his link to Jung, by introducing archetypal theory into his thinking, though he did not include anything explicitly like Jung's "Self" in his clinical considerations.

Langs' development of this approach to listening or, more precisely, to the process of listening-intervening-validating is, in this author's opinion, his seminal contribution to psychoanalysis. Nonetheless, we will see in the next two chapters that there are reasons for thinking Langs actually underestimates its value, by using it only within the relatively narrow confines of his own approach to adaptation. Once we examine Jung's articulation of adaptation, we will begin to see that this method of Langs can in principle be expanded.

Two Types of Derivative Communication

A final point central to Langs' clinical theory is his differentiation of two kinds of derivative communication, which he terms simply "Type One" and "Type Two" derivatives (Langs, 1978; Langs, 1979; Langs, 1982). This distinction differentiates derivatives according to their reference: Type One

---

12. This is all summarized in Langs (2004). Langs indicated to me in personal communications that he considered this way of listening to material to be his most important technical contribution, a point with which I agree.

derivatives are those which refer primarily to the patient's life outside the clinical setting, and Type Two derivatives are those which primarily comment on the clinical interaction. To the extent that we follow Langs' approach, the gold standard of unconscious communication is the Type Two derivative, because it is both an unconscious communication and it comments on the clinical process itself, thereby (1) potentially indicating to the therapist areas of unconscious conflict in the treatment and (2) guiding or validating the appropriate interventions for the therapist. The example in the previous section from Goodheart is an example of the Type Two derivative: though the patient offers a narrative on his business partner and their relationship, the derivative communication appears to be a commentary on what requires attention and potential correction in the therapy process itself.

Part and parcel of Langs' critique of the psychoanalysis of his time was that it focused, he claimed, on conscious-level material and, at best, Type One derivatives (i.e., unconscious communications referring exclusively to the extraclinical life of the patient [Grotstein, 1984]). For example, suppose the therapist in Goodheart's example was aware of a latent discomfort the patient had with talking directly to his wife about certain deficits in their relationship. In that case, the therapist might take the patient's story about his communicative difficulties with his business partner to be a disguised communication about his marital relationship and its specific challenges. In that case, the therapist would be interpreting the material as a Type One derivative, because the material is read in terms of the patient's life outside of therapy. Though such an interpretation can be valuable in some measure and may in fact be correct as far as it goes, it is not, for Langs, the most potent or valuable type of unconscious communication since it doesn't refer to the therapeutic interaction and thus cannot improve and enrich that relationship or its healing potential.

Langs underlines the understandable temptation on the part of the therapist to avoid interpreting unconscious material as Type Two derivative material, precisely because such an interpretation could highlight the patient's unconscious perception of the therapist's clinical errors, regarding either interventions or the mismanagement of the frame (Langs, 1978; Hodges, 1984). Consequently, there is always a tendency on the part of the therapist or analyst to allow countertransference resistances to influence their interactions with patients, by avoiding the potential Type Two meaning of unconscious materials. Nonetheless, it is right at this point, according to Langs, where the deepest analytic work can be done.

It is worth noting that Langs is less than perfectly clear on certain details surrounding his distinction between Type One and Type Two derivatives. For example, in some cases, Langs treats all derivative communications as if they can be read either of these two ways (Langs, 1982). In other cases, the distinction sounds like it refers to two different sorts of derivatives, rather than two ways of reading the same derivative material. The validity of this theoretical point is, however, mitigated, once we recognize that, in either case, our analytic listening should focus on what is potentially a Type Two derivative and that that is true whether the category refers to how we listen or to a specific type of derivative communication.

Critical Considerations of Langs' Theory of Unconscious Communication

Before we move on to a clinical illustration, it might be worthwhile to offer some critical considerations of Langs' understanding of unconscious communication, the Archimedean point, as it were, of his theory. Since we accept the bulk of what Langs articulates, these critical considerations will focus on what the theory leaves out more than on disputing its claims.

Though Langs emphasizes learning to hear and read derivatives in patient material, this method seems an ideal rather than something appropriate to every clinical situation. One reason for this is that, for Langs, such communication assumes a Type A or secured-symbolizing field which is often not present or not frequently present in a given treatment. One of the potential limits to the approach, therefore, concerns its general usability, even if it can be granted that it is a powerful approach. A further limitation is how much it requires the therapist or analyst to keep in mind, such as noting what communicative field the current work is in, what the themes and/or tone of the derivatives suggest, and, of course, which possible adaptive context is provoking the unconscious communications and psychic conflict in the first place.[13] Analysis is always extremely complex for the analyst, to be sure, but Langs' approach can leave one wondering how generally applicable it is, both because of the number of non-symbolizing patients we typically see and because of all that must be kept in mind on the part of the therapist.

Another concern is that this theory is deeply rooted in the concept of "talk therapy," in that it is language and elements of linguistic communication that are the focus of unconscious communication for Langs. In fact, it is not so much dreams and unconscious images per se that are emphasized in Langs' method as the *linguistic vehicles describing them*, the narratives *about* the dreams and images. It is, of course, one of the achievements of the psychoanalytic tradition that it recognizes the nuances of language and turns them into tools of analysis. Yet any competent analyst, Freudian or Jungian, will be well aware that *both* the images *and* their linguistic vehicles offer analytic material, that one cannot focus exclusively on the linguistic vehicles of analysis and expect to get an entire picture of the analytic situation. While there may be a certain greater emphasis on linguistic vehicles in the Freudian as compared to the Jungian tradition, in

---

13. Langs (1982) develops a very demanding intellectual process for the psychotherapist: on the one hand, a three-part "listening-intervening schema" and, on the other, a six-fold "observational schema."

Langs' case a historical, nuanced emphasis appears to become something of a caricatured exaggeration.

Thus, not only themes—which are basically the translation of images into language vehicles—or tones—which Langs attributes to the narrative, not to the images on which they are based—are ripe fields of unconscious communication. Images evoked in the therapist's psyche, verbal images embedded in non-narrative communications, metaphors expressed in the form of gestures and physical reactions, and many other such factors often harbor unconscious communications, even if not offered in a linguistic or narrative form. Indeed, in this clinician's experience, one often gains a better access to unconscious material when images are correlated to certain affective tonalities than one gets from the linguistic vehicles articulating them, often directly indicating worthwhile (non-intellectualized) associations and unconscious materials associated with emotional disturbance. In general, human thinking and the largely thought-based linguistic vehicles we use to describe experience are deeply influenced by formal logic and therefore tend to operate in terms of cause-effect or ground-to-consequent relationships, whereas feeling life bestows meaning according to similarity-and-difference relationships. For example, material with a certain disturbing affective tone often naturally feels related to some other experience with a similar affective tone. The previous experience does not cause the present one, but it does amplify the pain and conflict in part because it is similarly affectively toned to the current experience. Thus emotional life works not through causal-like or ground-to-consequent relationships, the basic form of relationship implicit in natural language use, but through a correlation of affective qualities. Yet oddly enough, even though "emotional disturbance" is the term Langs uses most frequently to describe psychic conflict, it seems as if his method skips over precisely where we find emotional disturbance most directly, which is not in the themes and tones of the derivatives but in the correlations between images and affective tonalities.[14]

Finally, Langs' approach, as we have come to expect, is very externally oriented, because he understands adaptation always as a reaction to external reality. We will later suggest that this is a one-sided approach and that it also carries with it a strongly intellectually toned approach to analysis, something which also buttresses the previous point. In many ways, Langs' approach reduces analytic work to gaining insight into the unconscious in order intellectually to formulate the psychic and emotional disturbances. But Langs does not seem to leave room for other approaches to

---

14. It might have further aided Langs' approach had he considered other variables in language. For example, language used in the form of an assertion—whereby someone posits some state of affairs—is quite a bit different from, say, language used declaratively, such as in a declaration of love to someone. The latter is not a merely statement of fact, as the first is, but in some sense "carries" and communicates the experience in the language. Differentiations of this kind are of prime importance for psychoanalytic forms of therapy but are rarely highlighted and lacking in Langs' otherwise subtle investigations.

the unconscious that are less intellectual, such as the use of reverie. Similarly, the kind of access to unconscious material that a strong feeling function can give, as when one is concerned directly with affective tone and the experience of value and value-conflict that a patient is having, is also non-existent in this approach.

Thus, though Langs' theory and practice is, in this author's view, deeply illuminating of unconscious realities and can be very successful when used well, both Langs' formulations and Langs' strongly intellectual and linguistic approach to analysis and therapy appear to be torsos of an analytic method, rather than the comprehensive method that Langs was attempting to develop.

Clinical Illustration

Clinical Example

To illustrate Langs' approach, I turn to a modified clinical example from early in my therapeutic career. The example focuses less on the patient's general psychological issues in treatment than on a specific problem related to a secure frame and communicative field and how Langs' approach was used to uncover the nature of the psychic conflict involved.

Bruce, a forty-two-year-old male, contacted me by email with the words "Anima problems" in the subject line. According to his email, Bruce was looking for a Jungian therapist and, as he forthrightly stated with a laugh in the opening session, he was looking for the "cheapest Jungian therapy" he could find. The precipitating cause was a set of problems he was having with some women coworkers, where he felt "for the first time in his life" that women did not like him, that he was unintentionally aggravating them, and he didn't understand how or why he was doing so. He also, at his first session, reported that he had lost his connection to his imagination: he was not dreaming or at least remembering dreams, not writing poetry, not doing anything imaginative, as he had for most of his adult life. Having developed the rational side of his personality in recent years, as part of a second profession he was pursuing, it seemed like he could not get his imaginative life back. As treatment continued, it turned out that an absent father, an alcoholic stepfather, and problems with "surrogate" fathers were at least as important for Bruce as the issues with women and other issues he raised at the outset. Bruce had been involved with lay Jungian organizations for many years and so explicitly wanted a Jungian therapist, but he also wanted to pay as little as possible.

Right from the first session, the issue of finding "cheap Jungian therapy" was a subject of exploration for us. For my part, I was early on in my analytic training, still a candidate, and had not even attained my counseling licensure at this point; hence, I was working for an agency and at a significantly reduced rate. The issue of the cost of therapy came up virtually right away because Bruce was going to pay the lowest end of a sliding scale at the agency I worked for at the time (forty dollars), yet he thought (implausibly) that even this was more than he could afford. He wanted to come, therefore, only every other week. After having discussed many of the issues with which he was dealing, I thought he should come weekly. I also discovered in the first session that he expected to be promoted in a couple of months and would be making a six-figure salary. I suggested he come weekly and, if for some reason that position did not pan out, we could make new arrangements. He wanted to do the opposite: come only every other week now and consider coming every week once he had the new job.

I felt there was an odd resistance here. Bruce had put forth a good deal of effort to find an inexpensive Jungian, working for well below the typical rate in the area and well within his current price range. Our rapport was good, and Bruce seemed to feel unusually comfortable and allied with me, even in the first session. Further, he would be making six figures in two to four months, an amount several times what my other patients at the agency made. What would make him so cautious or resistant to get into the process? Later in treatment, we would see his money issues as a surrogate symbol for value issues, associated with his devaluation of his own therapeutic process.

After discussing the importance of weekly therapy and finding him adamant about coming only every other week, I proposed something against my better judgment, namely, that he take a further, second reduction if he were willing to be recorded for supervision purposes—something I was required to do leading up to state licensure. I told him that I did not think having a recorder present was an optimal situation, but that I would offer it if he would, in turn, agree to come to therapy weekly. With the further reduction, he would pay a mere twenty-five dollars per session. I was in fact bluffing, hoping he would not take up the offer but rather understand my offer as highlighting how important weekly therapy was and then willingly pay the forty dollars. Instead, he called my bluff, agreed to come weekly, pay only twenty-five dollars per session, and have a recorder in the room.[15]

I was not happy with this resolution. I had some previous experience of recording patient sessions off and on over the years and I always noticed two things: (1) when I forgot to bring the recorder or when the batteries went dead (the tape recorder would make a noise at that point, so both patient and I knew it was dead), the rapport, the clinical material, and unconscious communications were invariably—and often significantly—better than usual; and (2) though the tape recorder was small and (one would think) easy to ignore, I noticed patients frequently looked toward it, right when they were talking about emotionally difficult issues, often leaving me with the impression that they were holding back *because* of the recorder. While it was clear to me that recording and listening to sessions helped *me* as a new

---

15. An additional relevant point for this case material is that the amount I was paid as a therapist was the same, no matter what the patient was required to pay.

clinician, experience had convinced me that taping sessions, minimally, inhibited at least some patients' communications and, maximally, was something
they experienced as harmful.

This was all in my mind when I offered this option to Bruce and was
why I hoped he would decline; at the same time, I had to live with the
consequences if he accepted it. It seemed to me that seeing him weekly was
more a gain than the loss of having the recorder in the room, despite my
objections to the latter. Through the first ten sessions, my decision seemed
justified. Above all, by the tenth session, Bruce was reconnecting to his
imagination and his unconscious: he was dreaming and remembering dreams
(for the first time in six years), and he seemed more vitalized and eager to
continue our work. My worries about the recorder diminished, and we
proceeded to a new phase of treatment. About this time, Bruce signed the
contract for his new job, which would take effect in another month or so.

Yet it was just at this point in treatment, just when a richer connection to
his imagination and his unconscious was getting established, that the recorder
began to loom larger in his psychological life. It felt as if the recorder had not
mattered so much for the first ten sessions, perhaps because the adaptive task
in those sessions was helping Bruce reconnect to his imagination and unconscious yet, once that reconnection had been established, the recorder became a
new adaptive problem. I first noted the issue a few sessions into this new phase
of treatment, when, as we worked a dream, Bruce suggested that maybe he
had some homosexual feelings toward a figure in his dream. Completely
unexpectedly, Bruce suddenly reached over to the recorder, picked it up, and
spoke into it with a mock serious tone, "It should be noted for the record and
by whoever is listening to this that I am *not* saying that I am a homosexual."
We both laughed at his humorous performance, but I was unsure which issue
to pursue: his concern at being perceived a homosexual or the way the recorder
was impacting his communication. Clearly there was an unarticulated fantasy
of someone listening in, perhaps someone imagined as a judge or moral figure,
given the pedantic tone and style of Bruce's pronouncement.

I decided to explore the homosexual anxieties, rather than the communication issue, but I kept the latter in mind for the future. Bruce denied ever
"really" having homosexual feelings and the issue was put to rest for the
moment. Since we had agreed to discuss the problem of the recorder once
his pay increased, I brought it up again in the next session. Bruce said, quite
irrationally I thought, he wasn't sure if he could "yet" afford a higher rate.
He asked, "Do I really have to go back and have my payment recalculated?"
in a tone which reminded me of my adolescent child asking if he *really* has
to take the garbage out today. I wasn't sure if this was subterfuge or if Bruce
had really forgotten that he had received *two* reductions: one, his rate being
lowest on the sliding scale and, the second, a further reduction below the bottom of the sliding scale because of the use of the tape recorder. I responded
by telling him that it was certainly the agency's expectation that he would
have the payments recalculated with his raise but that, from my standpoint,

I was less worried about the sliding scale adjustment than about the second reduction, born of having the recorder in the room. I reiterated the concerns I had mentioned in the opening session about the recording sessions and, knowing me better at this point, he knew how seriously concerned I was about it. Typical to him, he reverted to some humor and then said he would "think about it."

Bruce's communications from that session onward, however, took an interesting turn. From the beginning of treatment, Bruce frequently expressed contempt for people in authority, often with brief quips toward "bean counters" and the like. But for the next thirty-some sessions, the themes altered somewhat. Bruce now spoke about *nosy* supervisors, about how he hid things he did from his boss or employer or the government, about the various ways he had discovered getting around his bosses or around "The Man's" requirements, and so forth. As a rule, these comments were at best only obliquely related to the issues we might be speaking about and would seem often to emerge purely spontaneously, typically without any obvious connection to the current material.

Now Bruce happened to have had a number of "negative fathers" in his life and so I frequently explored this latter material, wondering if this change of theme in his material was related to his negative father complex, his memories of paternal abuse, and so forth. Yet, as a rule, this exploration yielded little further unconscious material—a point Bruce would note without my help, with comments like "nothing else is coming." On the other hand, when I took his comments on authorities less as emergent intrapsychic material about his father complex than as *adaptive* material triggered by the recorder being in the room, they made more sense: the themes of nosy supervisors, of authorities trying to find out what he was doing, and of getting around authorities, etc., appeared to be derivative communications about the tape recorder and they all indicated that, whatever Bruce's conscious stance, *unconsciously* he experienced recording his sessions as a violation, inhibiting his communication and his ability to access his unconscious material. If the tape recorder went dead, his body relaxed, and the sessions seemed freer and richer from the standpoint of unconscious material. I would in fact periodically loop his material back to the recorder interpretively, whenever the derivatives suggested the latter was provoking unconscious reactions, focusing both on the tape recorder itself and the self-esteem issues implied by his wanting therapy cheap to the point that it was reduced in quality. Bruce would seem to consider what I had to say carefully, promising to think about it, but avoiding doing anything in the direction of getting rid of the tape recorder.

We had a watershed moment in about the forty-fifth session. We were exploring experiences of various surrogate fathers in Bruce's life, when Bruce spontaneously recalled a male high school teacher he had not mentioned before. This teacher had taken an interest in Bruce and would bring him to concerts, cultural events, and the like. Bruce reported that he had thought at the time that the teacher could be the father he never had. After about six months, the teacher seduced Bruce and for about six months more they would frequently have sex. Bruce said he didn't like the sex, but at first felt that he had to agree to do it, since he was getting other benefits from this teacher; later he asked the teacher to stop, which the latter did.

As he spoke about this experience, it became clear that this was an emotionally significant time in Bruce's life yet, when I tried to help Bruce move into his feelings, his intellectual defenses increased: his tone became distant to the point of being cavalier, he spoke as if observing someone else from a distance, even making cynical fun of his younger self rather than contacting the old feelings. My own feelings intensified; indeed, I began to feel what I could only assume were his own anxiety, humiliation, and devastation, something which his memories seemed to provoke but which he could not entirely feel for himself—the phenomenon of the "interactive field" mentioned in chapter 1. Bruce continued with the cavalier tone, talking distantly—as Ogden would put it—*about* the pain at realizing that he was still without a father in his life and that he had only been a sex object to this teacher, but he could not speak *from* the pain.

If this interaction had been the entire session, I quite likely would have interpreted Bruce's pain and humiliation in terms of his individual trauma and father-longing—a largely intrapsychic interpretation. However, before I could make this intervention, Bruce began to say with a tone of relief that he had never told anyone this story before, but then caught himself, saying, "Well . . . I did tell one other person . . . but that didn't work out so well," his voice trailing off. I did not say anything but just looked at him, questioningly and expectantly. He then continued the story.

As a boy of six, living amid the unhappy relationship between his mother and alcoholic stepfather as well as further stresses from his abusive, sixteen-year-old half-brother living with them, Bruce had a breakdown in school. His mother took Bruce to a child psychologist, who saw him for a number of years; Bruce retained a good feeling about the psychologist. Twelve years later, when Bruce graduated high school, he wanted to get the sexual affair with his high school teacher off his chest and the only person he could think of with whom to do that was the child psychologist who, though retired, invited Bruce to talk with him. Bruce gave the psychologist a brief description of the issue on the telephone. The psychologist invited Bruce to his home and Bruce had lunch with both the psychologist and his wife (who had been the psychologist's secretary when the psychologist had been working). After lunch, the psychologist invited Bruce for a walk, rather than going back to his home office. They ended up a few blocks away, where the psychologist further invited Bruce into a private apartment he kept, unbeknownst to his wife. It turned out that this psychologist frequently brought children there for sex and asked Bruce then and there to have sex with him . . . Bruce declined.

Bruce remained largely cavalier and distant, even though I could see from the tenseness of his body and his moist eyes that he was trying with all his might to "hold it together." In the few minutes left in the session, I tried unsuccessfully to help him to enter his feelings. At the end of the session, I told him I thought we needed to explore this material in more detail, a point with which he agreed. I mentioned that he seemed rather cavalier in the telling, and he said that, "well, yes, it isn't easy to allow myself to feel all that again." I left it at that, and we parted. As Bruce went out the door, he shook my hand, which, up to that point he had rarely done and said, smiling sadly, "So . . . be gentle with me." I nodded.

I felt devastated for Bruce after he left. From an intrapsychic standpoint, it was clear that these two deeply violating events needed exploration. But I also recognized something else in these two stories of violation. The two stories were about boundary violations, violations of the frame by a trusted person in a power situation. The second story was about a "third party" (the psychologist) finding out about the first violation, a third party who was also a mental health professional intending to use the information to try to reviolate Bruce. Though he spoke with humor as he left, Bruce's call to be gentle indicated how costly it was for him to trust me and, implicitly, the third person who, I gathered from this derivative communication, was my supervisor, present in the consulting room through the tape recorder. How was Bruce to explore indescribably painful experiences when his therapist was acting like the teacher by "using" his material (e.g., for supervision) and while that anonymous mental health professional supervising me was also acting like the psychologist, voyeuristically listening in to Bruce's painful and private experiences, perhaps for some gains of his own? The derivatives strongly suggested that he unconsciously felt that both I and my supervisor were violating him anew.

I reflected on that session the entire week, always coming back to the same conclusion: the recorder was a frame violation which was retraumatizing my patient; both I and my supervisor were violating the patient by using his recorded material, I for supervision, my supervisor—in my patient's unconscious phantasy—for his own voyeuristic purposes. I therefore began the next session talking to Bruce about the recorder and what I thought occurred in the previous session, reiterating that I thought it would be in his best interests if we stopped recording his sessions entirely. Bruce's face—for the first time—seemed to express understanding of the issue. He said he would confer with his wife about the extra fifteen dollars per session, in order to be rid of the tape recorder. The next session began with us ritually turning the tape recorder off and exploring the material from the previous two sessions in detail.

As soon as we stopped recording, Bruce's entire attitude toward therapy began to change and his level of trust in me appeared to increase. The very session we removed the tape recorder, he began speaking of positive-themed narratives about care for his son, including loving, grateful narratives, as well as poignant recognitions and regrets over his failures, derivatives I interpreted as unconscious perceptions of how I had failed him by allowing the tape recorder in the room in the first place but also gratitude that I had fixed the situation by getting rid of it. For about a dozen sessions after, Bruce requested that he use the couch, thinking it might bring him into greater depths of the feeling from which he had been defending himself. Several previously forgotten or repressed memories came to the surface during those sessions, helping us understand some of the sources of many neurotic elements in Bruce's psychic life. When Bruce was not on the couch, he was relaxed and lost much of his stiffness. Whereas he had previously always sat up straight in the chair, once the tape recorder was gone he often began by loosening his tie, sometimes sitting sideways in the chair, sometimes taking off his shoes; he could cry and laugh, he recalled and faced the remembrance of a miscarriage his mother had of a baby that would have been his little brother; he could speak of his mother lovingly but also angrily, especially about how she did not defend him from the many male "monsters" who damaged him throughout his life. And he could begin to grieve the lack of father in his life and recognize how seeking that father had unconsciously determined so many decisions in his life. When treatment was cut short because he took a new job some hours away, he could break down a bit but also tolerate the recognition that one of the few males he had ever known who had always stayed with him, remained interested in him, and always did his best to listen to him, would be left far behind in that consulting room of the city he was leaving.

Summary

All five features of Langs' approach, outlined earlier, played a crucial role in this part of Bruce's treatment. Particularly important for this case were the changes in communicative style mentioned only cursorily in the final paragraph of the vignette, but which correlated in large measure to alterations in the transference relationship throughout the treatment.

Even in this small piece of the case, one can recognize the mutual adaptation, where we each had to understand something of each other and adapt in ways that often included confronting our own unconscious shadows, in order to work better together (e.g., my attitudes toward recording sessions and his feelings about the cost of therapy). The recorder itself, as the case material demonstrated, provoked both adaptive and specifically frame material, the presence of which inhibited the creation of the Type A/secured-symbolizing field and forced a maladaptive communicative relationship between us. This was so primarily because there was implicitly a third person in the room via the recorder, violating the basic assumptions of privacy and anonymity characteristic of the secured frame. Furthermore, the interpersonal communication was not the only thing inhibited here, but also Bruce's communication with his own unconscious life, thus limiting the extent to which valid and valuable unconscious communications were available. We can especially see the interactive nature of the therapy where I seemed to be holding Bruce's pain and devastation over his treatment at the hands of two trusted people, as well as some of his anxiety over being left alone with a mental health professional without the protection of a tape recorder. The stories about the violating teacher and violating psychologist could have been interpreted along the lines of Type One derivatives but by focusing on their potential Type Two meaning, they verified the problems associated with recording the sessions. Langs' adaptive model of unconscious communication and listening-intervening-validating were key in my understanding of the issues surrounding the tape recorder, such as the new narratives of paternal failures but loving relationships that confirmed the value of removing the tape recorder and the importance of fixing the frame. In this aspect of Bruce's treatment, the specific characteristics of Langs' method, with its focus on adaptation, a sufficiently secure frame, and analytic listening provided the basic framework for what success it attained.

Excursus: Final Phase: Adaptation and Death Anxiety

We mentioned earlier that one major difference appears in Langs' later work which does not have significant ramifications for *how* one works clinically but does have significant ramifications concerning *what* one is listening for. Over the first two decades of Langs' published work, he saw himself as modifying psychoanalytic theory rather than originating a new theory. Hence, he based his work on existing psychoanalytic literature, on the one hand, and his own clinical and supervisory experience, on the other. Beginning in the 1990s, his orientation changed, based on a changing understanding of adaptation: Langs came to believe that most people come to therapy because they are dealing with traumas and trauma-based emotional disturbances and therefore that adaptive contexts usually include trauma, death, and/or death-related anxieties. But Langs also found that psychoanalytic literature did little to elucidate this point, theoretically or clinically (Langs, 2004). Over time, Langs came to believe that, right from Freud's own metapsychological shift from the topographical theory (which was less about sex per se than about sex *trauma*) to the structural theory (which is really about sex), the psychoanalytic tradition had not only misunderstood but was actually in denial about the significance of trauma and especially death-related trauma, a denial which has burdened the psychoanalytic tradition since (Langs, 2010).

Consequently, Langs turned to other literatures in his quest to understand trauma and its meaning for patients. In his final theory, Langs posits that adaptation (as we noted in the chapter 1) is fundamentally a biological concept and only secondarily and by application a psychological concept. As such, if we are to understand the nature of adaptation properly, we need to extend the range of our knowledge beyond purely psychoanalytic or more broadly psychological literature, into biology and evolutionary theory. Langs' new theory led him to rearticulate his adaptive clinical theory into its final version, the "adaptive paradigm," based on the idea that psychic conflict is ultimately rooted in trauma and death anxiety. From the standpoint of clinical theory, this move does not greatly alter the style or method of Langsian practice, other than by highlighting the fact that death, trauma, and death-anxiety are assumed to be persistent triggers or adaptive contexts for psychic disturbances and conflicts.

From a theoretical standpoint, however, the alteration is somewhat more dramatic. For one, Langs opens himself up to a new kind of psychological theory, Jungian archetypal theory (Langs, 2010), by which he describes the fundamental structure of trauma and trauma-based emotional disturbances. Further, Langs develops the distinction mentioned previously, between the "unconscious" and the "deep unconscious," the former basically the same as the Freudian unconscious—a personal unconscious born of repressed and denied contents—the latter what Langs calls a "wisdom system," which illuminates the nature of a patient's psychological difficulties and traumas. It is the deep unconscious which provides clinical insight to help the patient: it is impersonal, includes a primitive ethical system based on death traumas, death anxiety, and the *talion* law, and communicates derivatively (Langs, 2004). Further, whereas Langs' earlier work lacked much by way of a theoretical exposition of the nature of the psyche, his later work includes a fairly comprehensive description of what he terms "the emotion-processing mind."

At the time of Langs' death, he had been working within this adaptive paradigm for over a decade and had been working toward it a decade prior to that. Those final twenty years of his professional life were challenging, because the changes in his theory led to crises in his practice and crises regarding his connection to the psychoanalytic world, both of which—according to his own account—were brought about by his insight that psychic conflict is rooted in death-related traumas and anxiety, something which, in the end, neither patients nor fellow analysts wanted to hear. Human nature, Langs came to believe, is something of a failure of the evolutionary process: on the one hand, those who survive and succeed in life are typically those who deny death and its concomitant anxieties; on the other, it is generally those same people who are the most pathological and who not only suffer but as a rule inflict the most suffering on others, precisely because they are not cognizant of their death-related anxieties. At the time of his death, Langs was working on a manuscript analyzing the American presidents, where he would show, among other things, how their individual traumas and death-related anxieties expressed themselves in the often pathological actions they undertook as presidents.

One doesn't have to be an expert in derivative communication to see that, whatever the value of these points for understanding psychoanalysis and larger issues in society, Langs' own suffering is also expressed in this

principle—especially his feeling that he was blacklisted from a largely unconscious psychoanalytic community, in part because he spoke the unspeakable
about death and death-related traumas and anxieties. These alterations in
the theory, however, do not fundamentally change Langs' understanding of
clinical practice, except by way of a new emphasis on what one listens for
and a new imperative that therapists always be aware of the various ways in
which traumas and death-related anxieties constitute the depth dimensions
of their own psyches, so that their natural denial of death does not skew
their work with patients.

Conclusion

We can formulate Lang's clinical theory schematically as follows.

(1) First, Langs' theory was not simply a meditation on clinical practice. It was instead produced by a set of clinical problems, problems which
were not always acknowledged by other theorists but which, for our purposes, I will simply assume were indeed problems. The first problem is one
of clinical practice: Langs believes that only by understanding the adaptive
task or trigger can one successfully interpret the nature of psychic conflict
and the specifics of unconscious communication in a patient, at least with
any certainty. It is possible that an analytic practitioner might have a good
intuition of what is happening or that the images of a dream or fantasy,
for example, might give direction to what is the likely trigger for adaptive
issues. But only on condition that one can recognize or at least have a good
hypothesis of the adaptive problem can an analyst expect to be able to
interpret, with some certainty, what especially the unconscious dimension
of the psychic conflict consists in. This point, it should be noted, derives
from the adaptive nature of the psyche, not because of any individual
predilections on the part of any given patient. Hence there is a theoretical
postulate underpinning this assumption of Langs' part, namely, that the
psyche seeks adaptation by nature, a point we emphasized in chapter 1.

(2) A second clinical problem, related but different from the first, is that
adaptation, for Langs, always has an inherently "external" orientation: it is
always in some measure a response to specific external stimuli. Since the psyche, on Langs' account, is by nature adaptive and since adaptation always
includes the external, situational element or environment, it follows that any
attempt to understand the unconscious sources of psychic conflict without
the consideration of the external trigger or adaptive context amounts to pure
intuition at best, a free association or speculation at worst, because one cannot understand an adaptively motivated unconscious communication if one
does not understand the external stimulus to which one is adapting. Hence
both understanding the nature of the adaptation at hand (point 2) and the
understanding of the patient's unconscious material (point 1) require understanding the (external) adaptive context or trigger.

(3) It follows from these two points that all sound clinical technique must have an adaptive component, at least to the extent that the clinical technique in question requires the recognition and interpretation of unconscious material. Consequently, one cannot validly interpret a supposed transference reaction on the part of the patient, without understanding what one may have done as a clinician to provoke the reaction and, ultimately, differentiating what aspect of the reaction might be adaptive (and thus rooted in a valid, unconscious perception) versus what might be maladaptive (and thus at least in part the fruit of pathological psychic factors). Similarly, one cannot validly interpret a dream without any notion of the external trigger to which the dream might be an adaptive reaction. On Langs' account, a dream is not merely a spontaneous psychic event but is also always an event which is motivated by adaptive issues of some kind. Material that seemingly emerges spontaneously from the unconscious, such as in the case material in this chapter, requires that one seek an adaptive motivation for it and, if possible, interpret it as a Type Two derivative. Without that adaptive motivation, we might think the patient's comments are merely reliving old father issues or simply demonstrative of a paranoid tendency, each of which might be true as well, but neither of which turned out to be the current, burning problem for the patient.

(4) Finally, the single most important and defining characteristic of Langs' thinking is his insistence on a specific way of listening to patient material. This way of listening can be characterized by three steps, on the part of the clinician: (1) listening to patient material adaptively, trying to pick out how the material and the adaptive task mutually illuminate each other: the core, one might say, of analysis proper; (2) offering interventions, primarily of an interpretive variety, based on this way of listening, thereby bringing to consciousness the unconscious material of which the patient is still unaware; and (3) listening again for the sort of material that this intervention brings up in the patient—the patient's adaptive response to the therapist's intervention—regarding its themes and/or tone, as a way of verifying the original listening and correlating intervention: listening-intervening-validating.

We will return to each of these points in the final chapter.

CHAPTER 4

Adaptation in Carl Jung

Introduction

More than Freud and the classical psychoanalysts prior to Hartmann, Carl Jung treats adaptation as a living part of both his clinical theory and his general conception of the psyche. Yet Jung's approach to each is by no means like that of Langs'. Langs, in part because he was a product of the reductive and materialist science of his time, seeks to find a single principle in terms of which everything else is to be understood; hence the primacy of adaptation for Langs and the language of the "adaptive paradigm." In contrast, Jung, though methodologically rigorous in his own way, resists the more reductive and materialistic trends in contemporary science and certainly avoids any reduction of psychic conflict and functioning to a single principle. Jung's approach is more properly phenomenological and hermeneutic (Brooke, 2015), whereas Langs models his approach on hard sciences with their emphasis on single variables. Jung's growing concern, especially in his later work, is collecting as rich a stock of psychological data as possible— to the point of examining areas your average classical psychoanalyst of his time wouldn't have touched, such as mystical, alchemical, occult, and parapsychological phenomena (such as UFOs)—and thus he countenances multiple variables and principles, in a way that Langs does not (and perhaps could not). Indeed, it is in part because of Jung's consistent expansion of psychological data and principles that his original conception of adaptation can easily get lost among the vast range of topics about which he writes.

Though adaptation is indeed a living part of Jung's theory of the psyche and his clinical theory, he has no distinct treatise on it and in certain respects he appears to underrate the importance of what he does say about adaptation. It will be one of the tasks of this chapter, therefore, to offer a coherent statement of his thought on adaptation and demonstrate just how significant it is for clinical practice, as well as offer some explanation of why Jung does not emphasize this aspect of his own work in the way one might expect.

The Concept of "Adaptation" in Jung

Unlike some ideas in Jung which underwent a number of transformations through time (such as the alterations in the notion that comes to be known as "archetypes" in his later work), Jung seems to retain a relatively consistent picture of adaptation throughout his work. Adaptation is specifically important in what we might call the "middle period" of Jung's work, from the time of his break with Freud in the early 1910s up to the late 1930s, when his interest turns much more to archetypal issues and alchemical studies. We will be concerned especially with his conception of adaptation in his essay *On Psychic Energy* (Jung, 1948).

On Psychic Energy, like many of Jung's works, was first published and then later "corrected" and republished. The editors of the English translation say that Jung began this essay just at the time of his break with Freud, but then set it aside until he had worked on the type problem (*Psychological Types*), after which time he completed and finally published it in 1928. The text went through further revisions and was both republished and retranslated, its republication in German occurring in 1948. These dates are important because they suggest both that Jung's thinking on these issues stretched the entire "middle period" of his work and that the final version most likely gained from the many papers on concrete clinical issues which he wrote during the 1930s, collected in volume 16 of the *Collected Works*, *The Practice of Psychotherapy*.

Before we turn to *On Psychic Energy*, however, we need to clarify a central interpretive issue regarding adaptation, namely, that Jung uses the term "adaptation" in two very different senses. These two senses are not only diverse from each other, but appear to be, in certain respects, *opposed* to each other, thus lending a good deal of confusion, actual and possible, to any discussion of adaptation according to Jung.

According to one sense of "adaptation," the term is primarily *descriptive*: it denotes a dynamic process characteristic of the human psyche, one which Jung poses in terms of the "progression and regression of libido (or psychic energy)" (Jung, 1948). This is the primary and what I will call the "dynamic" meaning of adaptation in Jung, because it refers to a basic dynamism of the psyche. It is also the sense of adaptation that correlates to the one we set forth in chapter 1 of this study and thus will be our primary interest in this chapter. A second acceptation of "adaptation," however, is not *descriptive* but *evaluative* (i.e., it is a value term indicating something negative or problematic, based on a person's relative identification with a collective or, in other words, with a person being too "collectively minded"). In contrast to the first meaning, this second meaning does not denote a basic or essential characteristic of the human psyche, but a purely factual (as opposed to structural) and contingent characteristic of a given psyche, defined by that person's unconscious identification with a social collective.

I will refer when necessary to this second term as the "collective sense" of adaptation, in contrast to the "dynamic sense" of the term.

It should be clear that these are two different meanings of adaptation and are distinct both conceptually and phenomenologically. Adaptation in the dynamic sense refers first of all to a consistent structural feature or tendency of the psyche and to its correlating process; the collective sense of adaptation, in contrast, refers to a contingent state of mind, not to a dynamism or to a process. Furthermore, it makes perfect sense to speak of someone as "too adapted," a common trope in Jungian literature, only if we mean the second sense of the term, precisely because the latter is a contingent and (conceived of as) a largely negative state of mind, suggesting a lack of differentiation from collective attitudes. It would, in contrast, make no sense to say that someone is "too adapted" in the first sense, because the term is being used to describe a basic psychic dynamism which occurs essentially and willy-nilly, not a contingent state: the psyche is adaptive by nature, quite independent of the question of how collectively minded an individual is. Consequently, one cannot be "too adapted" in that sense; to say so would be like saying that "the will is too volitional," as if it is too much what it is by nature. The dynamic meaning of adaptation, as I pointed out, is not evaluative but descriptive; the collective meaning is evaluative and in a negative sense. The first pertains to a natural and intrinsic psychic process, the second to a contingent even if habitual attitude. Since the first refers to an innate psychic dynamism and, thus, must in some way express the psyche's teleology, adaptation in that first sense must in principle be an aspect of the movement toward individuation. The second, collective sense of adaptation, in contrast, is typically inimical or at least a hindrance to individuation, because it suggests that one has lost some measure of the consciousness of one's distinctive personality and its teleology, in favor of the collective.

As helpful as these phenomenological and conceptual distinctions may be for differentiating these two meanings of adaptation, however, it is important that we not miss the deeper difference of principle. As we will see, adaptation in the first, dynamic sense of the term is actually right at the heart of any analytic process, as it is conceived within classical analytical psychology. This is so because adaptation in the dynamic sense is ultimately expressive of what Jung conceives of as the basic individuating function of the unconscious, namely, its *compensatory function* (Jung, 1953).[1] As we will try to show, adaptation in the dynamic sense occurs when unconscious processes are activated and provoked by adaptive demands. These demands are often experienced as if they are "orchestrated" by what Jung calls the "Self"—by what we might in fact, borrowing a term from the philosopher Hegel, call the "cunning" of the Self. These demands require a person to activate unconscious dimensions of their psychic functions, often against habitual avoidance as well as

---

1. I am grateful to August Cwik for underlining, in an earlier draft, how central the compensatory function of the unconscious is for the argument I am making.

projection and other defenses, in order to act in accordance with the call to individuation. Consequently, adaptation in the dynamic sense is a structural feature of the psyche, and its process is essentially bound up with personal transformation and individuation.[2]

In contrast, adaptation in the collective sense, as a rule, does not denote a development of greater consciousness or a movement toward individuation, since—again, as a rule—it is typically a development in the direction of unconscious identification with collective attitudes and mores. (I say "as a rule" in order to allow for the possibility that the individuation of some patients might actually *require* becoming a little more "collectively minded" in a certain sense—though even here, the call would not be to become more *unconscious* but rather to become more *conscious* of one's relationship to meaningful communities of various kinds.[3]) Furthermore, the development of a healthy persona also requires something of collective mindedness, yet again in a conscious, rather than unconscious, way.[4] Nonetheless, in most cases, adaptation in this second sense, outside of developing a healthy and conscious persona, hinders individuation, in that it leads to greater unconsciousness. Hence this is not only a different meaning of adaptation; it is, in a certain sense, an opposite to adaptation in the dynamic sense, since it denotes an attitude detrimental to the individuation process, whereas the dynamic sense of adaptation denotes an aspect of the basic drive within the psyche toward individuation.

Our primary concern will be with what we have called the "dynamic" sense of adaptation. This distinction between the meanings of the term will come up again later in the chapter. For current purposes, it is important that we keep the distinction in mind and recognize that what might be said of adaptation in one sense might well not apply to the other.

On Psychic Energy

Jung intended *On Psychic Energy* to be something of a definitive statement of certain aspects of his psychological theory, a point made evident by his insistence that he is correcting misinterpretations of his basic theory of the psyche and by his situating his understanding of the psyche and psychic energy in terms of broader scientific claims and laws of energy. It is in many respects Jung's most definitive statement on adaptation,

---

2. Stein's work (1998) can be seen as an attempt to articulate and illustrate this dynamic meaning of adaptation, especially in the second half of life.

3. Jung's discussions of these issues are a bit too undifferentiated to make this point easily, since he seems to conflate collectivity and community frequently. In our usage of the terms (which may not correspond exactly to Jung's) a collective is group joined largely through unconscious processes, whereas a community proper is a group united through largely conscious commitments and values.

4. My thanks to an anonymous reviewer for emphasizing the importance of this second sense of adaptation at least for persona development.

outlining his mature reflections on the nature of the psyche in general and adaptation in particular.

Adaptation dominates a specific section of this essay, where Jung attempts to understand how psychic conflicts arise. Jung also attempts to illustrate adaptation in terms that are quite different from those of Langs. One ground of difference is that Langs treats adaptation almost exclusively in clinical theory—at least prior to the last phase of his work—whereas Jung treats adaptation from the start in terms of a theoretical conception of psychic energy. Also, Langs tends to treat adaptation as a state to be achieved, whereas Jung's conception concerns adaptation as an ongoing process. Furthermore, Langs tends to treat adaptation as a problem of discrete external events which become clinically relevant. In contrast, Jung treats adaptation less in terms of a specific event or problem than in terms of broad trends of psychic development and especially in terms what Jung calls "psychological types."

This last point bears some clarification. Perhaps due to popularized versions of the Myers-Briggs system of classification as much as to anything else, Jung's "psychological types" are often construed as *personality* types, where "personality" suggests something like a cluster of innate traits. In contrast, Jung posits the types in terms of how one relates to one's environment; hence, if anything, the types represent not static traits but dynamic modes of adaptation. Jung is explicit about this in his 1923 lecture "Psychological Types" where he writes, "The conscious psyche is an apparatus for adaptation and orientation, and consists of a number of different psychic functions. Among these we can distinguish four basic ones: *sensation, thinking, feeling, intuition*" (Jung, 1923: para. 899; italics in original). It is therefore Jung himself who links the notion of psychological types to adaptation and even describes the types as modes of adaptation.

This point should not be lost on us, especially with regard to clinical practice, because the application of typology in clinical settings evidently requires not that we find some abstract type the patient supposedly exemplifies but that we discover a patient's dominant modes of adaptation. In practice, a patient's supposed "traits" can actually be quite different from the modes of adaptation the patient utilizes. This in fact can become quite a complicated business in clinical practice, as, for example, when a person seems to have a dominant form of adaptation when their public persona is operative versus those modes of adaptation more typical when the patient is at home and the persona less dominant. Or again, a patient might, from the standpoint of personality tendencies, be an "introverted intuitive feeler" but, because of education and work habit, tend to adapt publicly in terms of extroverted thinking or sensation. Differences of this sort, in fact, are often seen in the consulting room and are themselves frequently sources of psychological conflict and adaptive challenges for the patient. It is therefore important in clinical practice that one not jump too quickly to the conclusion of a patient's dominant psychological type.

It is also worth underlining that these four basic types Jung delineates are multivalent and thus denote a range of functioning; again, these are not static categories or singular modes of functioning but descriptive of diverse kinds of functioning which admit of many subspecies.[5] For example, the "thinking function" is used quite differently, say, in a process of free association or reverie from how it is used when one is coolly taking a distance to understand some difficult situation or when one is writing a paper on a topic one passionately believes in. Each of these cases includes the operation of the thinking function and in each case the thinking function might be being used well and adaptively: no single use of a function defines it so much that some other use of it might not just as well represent an aspect of that function. Since no function consists in one exclusive form of operation, typology must be used clinically with some caution and a good deal of nuance. The tendencies to reify psychological types in terms of personality categories and to treat the range of any given personality in simplistic categorial terms have unfortunately plagued the practical use of the types throughout its history.[6] These latter tendencies in some practitioners are quite possibly why Hartmann considered Jung's delineation of the types to be a "crude" analysis of adaptation, whereas the crudeness appears to be less in the types than in how and in how well they are used by any given clinician.

Given the importance of typology for Jung's understanding of adaptation, we can see why he set aside his work on adaptation to work first on the type problem, as the English editors and translators of *On Psychic Energy* mention.[7] Jung is straightforward about typology describing modes of adaptation in *On Psychic Energy* and, in this respect, he further differentiates his thought from that of Langs. For Jung, adaptation is virtually never about a singular, externally induced psychological problem or conflict in need of a solution, as it appears to be for Langs. Rather, adaptation is always in some measure about more lasting attitudes, stances, and orientations in the person. By posing adaptation in terms of internal, psychological type rather than external conflict, Jung articulates what is in principle a more properly psychological reason for conflicts associated with adaptation than Langs does. In the final analysis, the problem of adaptation for Jung is the problem of how a person develops and expands general psychological resources and energy through

---

5. My thanks to Mark Winborn for highlighting this point in reactions to an earlier draft of this work.

6. Sometimes Jung is implicitly or explicitly criticized for dealing theoretically with "pure types" when in practice the types are intermingled (e.g., Jarrett, 1988). However, it should be noted that this is in general an issue in the human sciences, namely, that one has to use what Weber terms "ideal types" in order to understand the nature of the range of deviant forms of the type.

7. It is important to mention the work of John Beebe, among English-language Jungians, who has done a good deal to illuminate the nature of the types. See especially his recent book (Beebe, 2017).

adaptive conflicts (adaptive process), rather than primarily about the concrete conflict and what one does to make it conscious and resolve it (state of being adapted). For this reason, Jung's discussions are less about specific external adaptations and more about internal, long-term changes (i.e., the movement toward individuation and wholeness) sometimes caused but always in part occasioned by external adaptive conflicts.

Theoretical Assumptions

Some understanding of the basic theoretical assumptions outlined at the beginning of *On Psychic Energy* bear upon Jung's discussions of adaptation and so must be summarized here. First, Jung introduces a way of understanding psychic energy in this essay which both relates it to and distinguishes it from other kinds of life energy. Psychic energy is first and foremost vital energy (i.e., the energy of organic life), an energy which Jung treats as a phenomenon which is not reducible to other kinds of energy. These claims are very much in keeping with continental European thinking of the time, especially of the phenomenological variety, where organic life demonstrates characteristics unlike purely physical forms of causality and thus must be treated as a phenomenon *sui generis*. We saw in chapter 1 how Jung marshals ancient arguments first systematized by St. Augustine to prove just this point, namely, that the soul is real and yet has a form of reality which is not material.

Furthermore, Jung argues that psychic energy is finalistic or teleological, presumably emphasizing this point against many practitioners of the psychological sciences in the 1930s who reduced psychic or organic reality to purely material principles. To say that psychic energy is "teleological" is among other things to say that the psyche is purposeful, that "it" does things and that "its" movements are meaningful. Hence Jungian practice is less about particular conflicts and their resolution than about learning why and how that conflict might be conducive to the growth and expansion of our experience of life, wholeness, and individuation. Jung explicitly considers adaptation—in the dynamic sense—a teleological concept, without which any theory of psychological development is impossible (Jung, 1948: para. 42).

A further aspect of Jung's concept of psychic energy is that it is *quantitative* in nature, which is to say that when we consider psychological change in our patients, we are raising, among other things, the question of "how much?" energy is located where.[8] For example, how much energy is being expended in this part of one's personality versus that part? This point is crucial for interpreting adaptation in Jung's sense, because he focuses less on an external adaptive context and more on the question of how that psychic conflict requires a different distribution of the quantum of psychic energy. In

---

8. Though one might be troubled by the spatial metaphor of "location" used for these discussions, virtually any differentiation of psychic reality uses such spatial metaphors (e.g., the "topographical" model of Freud).

fact, it should be clear already at this point that, if we understand adaptation in such terms, adaptation has the character of an operationalizing of teleology (i.e., the measure of the development and expansion of one's resources for adaptation is also a measure of the extent to which wholeness and individuation are progressing, since adaptational conflicts characteristically force the emergence of hitherto unconscious or at least latent psychic potentials). Precisely the value of adaptational conflicts, for Jung, is that they potentially expand the range of available conscious energy.

This quantitative conception needs to be utilized carefully in clinical practice. Jung is clear that the psyche must be conceived as a *relatively* and not *absolutely* closed system. When we work clinically, therefore, we can assume *prima facie* that, if some quantum of libido—Jung's term for psychic energy generally, not exclusively sexual energy (Jung, 1956)—is not where it once was in the personality then, all things being equal, it must be located somewhere else in the personality (e.g., when energy is displaced from the conscious personality to the unconscious or vice versa during some process of development). This quantitative notion is misused, however, if utilized as a principle of inference rather than a *prima facie* tool for understanding psychological change in a concrete patient. For example, certain versions of typology might infer that "*since* one is a thinker, one must not be a feeler," as if the presence of conscious energy in one function implies a necessary lack of energy in its opposite. This is an invalid use of the quantitative nature of psychic energy in Jung. The psyche is not an absolutely closed system; hence there is always the further option in principle that more energy has been drawn into conscious adaptive functioning from the unconscious and that the person therefore has developed both functions. Indeed, if the adaptive process works in the way it is meant to, according to Jung, the psyche *must* draw unconscious libido into the conscious system, since adequate adaptation consists among other things, in the enhancement of the availability of energy by introducing more consciousness into underused functions. The teleology of the psyche toward expansion and differentiation of psychic energy implies that the more one responds adequately to adaptive challenges, the more the psyche can draw energy from unconscious or from hitherto unassimilated sources of energy as necessary. Hence—and this is a further point—the more individuated or whole the person, the less one can make such typological inferences from the presence of energy in one function to the lack in its opposite, precisely because the inference assumes a scarcity or limited range of possible energy (i.e., that it is an absolutely, rather than relatively closed system). In Jung's theory there is always an "excess of libido" stored unconsciously, which is what makes possible the canalization of libido and, in principle, the development of human culture (e.g., Jung, 1948: para. 91). For these and other reasons, one must avoid invalid assumptions or inferences of energy scarcity in interpreting Jung's quantitative notion of psychic energy.

Nonetheless, within the boundaries of a relatively closed energic system, we can say, with Jung, that there is—*prima facie*—a principle of equivalence in the psyche, such that when we see a lack of expected energy in one place, we are likely to find that that energy has moved to another location in the psyche and, often, we see some sort of movement of energy between conscious and unconscious and back again. Such moves are often short-term changes, however, because, assuming a movement toward wholeness is largely successful, the long-term movements should result in an expansion in the overall quantum and differentiation of energy available to consciousness, not merely the displacement of existing energy.

Posing adaptation in terms of energy displacement and in terms of a relatively rather than absolutely closed system is a central contribution to the theory of adaptation and potentially provides something missing from Langs' theorization, in that Jung's interpretation of adaptation in terms of energy underlines that a psychologically adequate adaptive response not only heals conflict but *adds psychic resources to conscious life*. This approach therefore helps to underline how something is gained for the psyche in a lasting way, beyond the immediate resolution of outer adaptive problems.

Progression and Regression of Libido

According to Jung, progression of the libido occurs to the extent that one "satisfies the demands of environmental conditions" (Jung, 1948: para. 61) or, in other words, is adapted to those conditions. At this point, there is no fundamental difference between Jung's and Langs' conception of adaptation. However, Jung also thinks that adaptation is defined by two elements: "(1) the attainment of an attitude" and "(2) the completion of adaptation by means of that attitude" (Jung, 1948: para. 60), the underlying premise being that adaptation challenges the *range* and *quantum* of available psychic energy. The normal course for the psyche is to respond and to adapt to a given situation without conflict. However, new adaptational challenges can result in one either failing to have the energy available to consciousness or failing to have the energic resources in a form conducive to successful adaptation, according to psychological type, forcing conflict as well as a new kind of adaptation. Jung offers a somewhat schematic but nonetheless telling example:

Jung imagines a patient whose natural tendency is to adapt through the feeling function. This patient is now confronted with an adaptive challenge or situation for which the range of functioning typical to feeling is inadequate: the patient must activate a largely unconscious and underused thinking function in order to adapt to the new situation, because the dominant feeling function cannot resolve the adaptive challenge. Jung writes:

> In this case the feeling-attitude breaks down and the progression of libido also ceases. The vital feeling that was present before disappears, and in its place the

psychic value of certain conscious contents increases in an unpleasant way; subjective contents and reactions press to the fore and the situation becomes full of affect and ripe for explosions. These symptoms indicate a damming up of libido, and the stoppage is always marked by the breaking up of the pairs of opposites. During the progression of libido the pairs of opposites are united in the co-ordinated flow of psychic processes. Their working together makes possible the balanced regularity of these processes, which without this inner polarity would become one-sided and unreasonable. (Jung, 1948: para. 61)

Jung here analyzes the adaptive situation in terms of an imbalance in the patient's psychological typology. The experience of adaptive conflict arises because, on the one hand, the outer situation requires something beyond what the psychic resources present in the patient's dominant psychological type can offer and, on the other, because the patient cannot seem to marshal sufficient psychic energy to activate the other, opposing but complementary function. Successful adaptation is analyzed in terms of a coordination of the distinct types of adaptation—the psychological types—especially those which Jung considers opposing types, such as feeling and thinking or intuition and sensation, working together. In this situation, the patient experiences the adaptive conflict based on an unactualized and hence partially unconscious thinking function. In such a situation, as Jung suggests, there is a growing affect, "affect" being the term Jung uses in this case for an excess of emotional energy, usually expressed as some sort of frustration, due to the inability to resolve the adaptive challenge by means of the dominant typology (Jung, 1923).[9]

As Jung formulates it:

Hence it is essential for progression, which is the successful achievement of adaptation, that impulse and counter-impulse, positive and negative, should reach a state of regular interaction and mutual influence. This balancing and combining of pairs of opposites can be seen, for instance, in the process of reflection that precedes a difficult decision. But in the stoppage of libido that occurs when progression has become impossible, positive and negative can no longer unite in co-ordinated action, because both have attained an equal value which keeps the scales balanced. (Jung, 1948: para. 61)

Hence, a balance of consciousness in terms of a successful balancing of psychological types, especially opposing types, allows for successful adaptation, even where, in any given situation, one of the functions may and indeed must take the lead (so the scales are never perfectly balanced). But even in that situation, the one function leads in a way that does not repress the opposing side and includes the coordination of each side with the other.

We can see here, in Jung's example, the compensatory function of the unconscious at work (Jung, 1948; Jung, 1953). For Jung, neurosis always

---

9. "Affects usually occur where adaptation is weakest, and at the same time they reveal the reason for its weakness, namely, a certain degree of inferiority and the existence of a lower level personality" (Jung, 1959: para. 15).

in some measure arises from one-sidedness, from a conscious stance so dominated by one attitude or typology that one cannot activate different or opposing typological functions (Jung, 1923). The unconscious, by virtue of its innate teleology toward wholeness and by virtue of the Self's attempt to bring balance to the conscious attitude, evokes a compensatory shift in consciousness. Because of this innate teleology, one is often left with the peculiar feeling of a kind of "providential" movement, a mysterious "forcing of the issue" that seems to entail that one react by activating hitherto unconscious dimensions of the psyche.[10] At times, one can stubbornly resist this movement, insisting that one will resolve the adaptive issue in the old way. Jung suggests that no matter how much one may attempt to resist its impulses, however, teleology and the compensatory balancing work of the Self will not allow one to rest, until the underused function and at least some of the shadow material associated with it is dealt with and managed.

It is worth considering for a moment one of the marks of the adaptive situation for Jung, what he describes in the earlier passage in the following terms: "The vital feeling that was present before disappears, and in its place the psychic value of certain conscious contents increases in an unpleasant way; subjective contents and reactions press to the fore and the situation becomes full of affect and ripe for explosions" (Jung, 1948: para. 61). This passage describes a quite typical situation in which adaptive issues arise. Two qualifications, however, might be illuminating. First, Jung uses the term "affect" in very precise way. For Jung, affect is always a kind of inappropriate emotional energy, such as this passage for example describes in terms of too much affect (Jung, 1923; Jung, 1959). It is worth highlighting, however, that the inappropriate affect may consist not only in too much emotional energy around an adaptive situation but also too little. It is easy enough to imagine a case where an adaptive context demands a response, yet the patient, rather than feeling frustration, for example, feels paralyzed, numb, or unable to react at all. While, in such a case, there is often a strong defense against feeling the pent-up affect, there are also cases, it would appear, where one is emotionally paralyzed by the adaptive demands, perhaps through years of habitually shutting down when a highly charged adaptive demand arises. Hence, in many cases, the inappropriate affect Jung speaks of may not be indicated through too much affect but rather indicated through too little: it is as if all emotional energy drains from conscious life into the unconscious. Indeed, Bruce's lack of affect as he first told the story of his teacher and then the child psychologist—which later oscillated to the opposite situation of him experiencing more affect than he alone could hold—were original indicators that a powerful adaptive issue was at stake, even before pent up energy later appeared.

---

10. Jung suggests that the reason there are multiple modes of adaptation (functions and attitudes) is that we are meant to activate all of them in order to relate fully to objects. See Jung, 1948: para. 28.

Furthermore, this issue of "appropriate" versus "inappropriate" affect should not be lost on us because it indicates something we saw in both Freud's and Hartmann's understanding of adaptation, namely, *an implicit value ranking*. Affect counts as too much or too little, presumably, because one has something of a value measure in mind, by which one judges too much or too little. Once again, lurking in the background of a theory of adaptation is some kind of value ranking or hierarchy which implicitly "demands" a certain response and by which we measure the extent to which a patient has adequately or inadequately responded. So far as I know, Langs does not even implicitly mention this value phenomenon, though it is evidently presupposed for Freud, Hartmann, and Jung. As we will see in moment, the issue of inappropriate affect will need to be distinguished from what Jung calls the "feeling function" which, while including certain emotional qualities that parallel what Jung means by "affect," has more of an objective relationship to the world than affect.

The quoted passages in Jung also highlight the importance of *regression* of the libido—a regression, it should be emphasized, which is not a regression to previous stages of development, as in Freud, but a regression of *energy* into the unconscious in the service of adaptive progression. In the earlier passages, the patient finds that the dominant trend of adaptation cannot work and, thus, an emotional and psychological regression in the form of the rise and intensification of affect and conflict occurs, indicated by unconscious psychic material pouring into consciousness (Jung, 1948: para. 61). This sort of "regression" amounts to a demand that the person adapts through using an underused function, something the patient experiences as primitive because the function is, in fact, underdeveloped. Nonetheless, by responding to this demand, the energy regressing into the unconscious can be transformed into new conscious energy, to be used for further development toward individuation and further progression of libido, leading to a less conflictual relationship to one's environment.

At this juncture, one further point relevant to our previous analyses is worth mentioning. There is a striking *parallel* between Jung's articulation of the adaptive process and the teaching of Hartmann. As we saw previously, Hartmann considered there to be four goals of adaptation, all of which he formulates in terms of equilibrium: (1) equilibrium of person and environment; (2) equilibrium among instinctual drives; (3) equilibrium among psychic functions ("mental institutions"), that is, a kind of structural equilibrium; and (4) equilibrium between the ego's own "synthetic function" (i.e., the ego insofar as it is a *force* of equilibrium) and the rest of the ego. While Hartmann poses these four kinds of equilibrium understandably in standard ego-psychological rather than Jungian language, each of the equilibriums he refers to seem to be expressed in Jung's approach. The adaptive process, according to Jung, arises when adaptive issues throw the equilibrium of person and environment off (number 1) and demands that the ego find the balance or equilibrium (number 4) through modifying the conscious-unconscious relationship (number 2) as well as modifying psychological functions (number 3), which for Jung would mean a rebalancing according to type. Though Hartmann in his essay describes Jung's typological analysis as "crude," Jung's analysis appears to express virtually the same points as Hartmann's analysis.

Langs and Jung

As should be clear enough at this point, Jung's approach to adaptation is quite different from Langs and not all the ways in which they are different can be treated of in this chapter without taking us far afield. Nonetheless, some level of comparison and contrast will help bring into focus both what Langs and Jung hold in common and where their differences from each other might produce a larger synthesis and where not.

One major difference between Langs and Jung is, as we pointed out in chapter 3, that Langs tends to understand adaptation exclusively in terms of external reality, whereby an adaptive task in the environment produces psychic conflict for a patient, which in turn requires an adaptive response. Jung's approach, in contrast, tends to focus on the external adaptive context only to the extent that it produces an internal issue which must be resolved. This understanding of the adaptive situation allows Jung to formulate what we might term a "cyclical" model of adaptation, one which moves along the following description: an outer adaptive context or trigger (in Langs' terms) occasions an internal, psychological conflict, born of the fact that the normal course of energy through the patient's dominant function (or functions) is inadequate to solve the adaptive problem smoothly; this situation in turn evokes an intensification (or excessive lack) of affect—which is to say a damming up of libido or psychic energy—which in turn requires the activation of hitherto unconscious or underused function(s) at a conscious level to resolve the external, adaptive problem. Hence, the external adaptive context requires an internal (i.e., intrapsychic) change, in order that that context can be resolved or at least resolved enough no longer to produce psychological conflict. There is therefore not only an *external* adaptive context, but an *internal* adaptive context, in that one must activate an underused psychic function. Once the latter is achieved to some extent, the external adaptation can in principle occur, because of the addition of new psychic resources in the form of the activation of the previously underused psychological function; solving the internal problem releases energic resources to solve the external problem. Adaptation to the outer requires adaptation to the inner and vice versa:

> By activating an unconscious factor, regression confronts consciousness with the problem of the psyche as opposed to the problem of outward adaptation. It is natural that the conscious mind should fight against accepting the regressive contents, yet it is finally compelled by the impossibility of further progress to submit to the regressive values. In other words, regression leads

to the necessity of adapting to the inner world of the psyche. (Jung, 1948: para. 66)

Thus, three important differences between Langs and Jung emerge at this point. First, Jung's conception of adaptation appears to be more complex than that of Langs. Langs' notion of adaptation would count as "one-sided" to Jung, because it is focused exclusively on a singular, linear relationship, such that psychic conflict and resolution is the dependent variable and the (external) adaptive problem the independent variable. That is in fact a necessary part of Langs' theory, because he insists that adaptational issues are "external," whereas psychodynamics is purely "internal." There is therefore no way to avoid this one-sidedness theoretically. In contrast, Jung conceives of adaptation in terms of multiple and cyclical relationships, in that external adaptive contexts produce psychic conflict, which in turn produces internal adaptive contexts, the resolution of which alone can resolve the outer context by means of an expansion of internal psychic resources. Thus, adaptation, for Jung, is always *simultaneously* an inner and an outer phenomenon or, to put it in Langsian language: there are always two, interrelated "adaptive contexts," an external and an internal. Indeed, in any given case, the outer or the inner could actually be the dominant source of conflict at any point in treatment, as in the example of anxiety over doing taxes offered in chapter 3. The sharp differentiation between "intrapsychic" and "adaptive" or between "psychodynamics" and "adaptation to external reality" on which Langs predicates much of his theory is foreign to Jung, for whom inner and outer adaptations are inherently and by an inner necessity connected.[11]

Second, Langs' treatment of adaptation focuses on discrete events of immediate import and how those adaptive contexts illuminate unconscious material which, as a rule, *also* pertain to immediate interventional contexts. Jung's treatment of adaptation, in contrast, focuses on how external adaptive contexts cause a second and, more importantly, *attitudinal* adaptive context, where relatively lasting dimensions of the personality are experienced in conflict and relatively lasting change of the personality demanded. In this respect, Jung's treatment underlines not only and not primarily the interventional contexts for the therapist but an ongoing *direction of change* to which a patient's psyche is inviting the patient and of which the analyst must be conscious not only as an immediate interventional context but as a long-term interventional orientation. In this respect, the Jungian analyst will generally interpret dynamic adaptation as indicative of movements of the Self, rather than as a purely factual need on the part of a patient to change in a given external adaptive context, because

---

11. Jung writes that, "No adaptation can result without concessions to both worlds. From a consideration of the claims of the inner and outer worlds, or rather from the conflict between them, the possible and the necessary follows . . . the *union of opposites through the middle path*" (1953).

the former would be read as a compensatory movement toward wholeness and individuation.

Third, as a consequence of Jung's analysis, we have to draw the conclusion that adaptive problems are never simply an immediate problem for resolution by means of insight and choice. Rather, Jung's orientation throughout his analysis of adaptation suggests that adaptive contexts pertain to long-term psychological reorientation, something that in practice Langs never treats of (though we cannot infer for that reason it was of no interest to him). In other words, Langs' clinical approach nearly always focused on what the *immediate* meaning of an adaptive context was, something his many clinical vignettes suggest over and over again. Jung, in contrast, does not focus on immediate adaptive issues, except as they provoke questions about typological and attitudinal change and therefore how a concrete adaptive issue relates to the overall development of personality. For this reason, one might draw the surprising conclusion that adaptation is, in a certain respect, more important for clinical practice for Jung than it is for Langs, though Langs speaks of it in virtually all his publications and Jung does not. The "greater importance" we are attributing to adaptation for Jung is not due to the quantity of ink he spent on but on the *level of change* he emphasized. Wholeness or individuation for Jung refers to how unconscious dimensions of the personality as a whole require activation, not only to the extent that one can obtain an immediate resolution to adaptive problems.

However, more important than the question of who thought adaptation was more important is the fact that, because of the differing levels of discussion of adaptation in Langs and Jung, their ways of thinking could in principle be complementary to each other. That is to say, Langs' emphasis was on the immediate needs of the patient to resolve adaptive problems and how clinical material posed those problems concretely. Jung recognizes the concrete adaptive issues ("adaptive context") but immediately moves to a broader level of orientation in the personality. There is no reason at this point to think therefore that these two approaches need be inimical to each other. Since they speak of different levels of psychic reality, the one the punctual present, the other the habitual, they should in principle be able to be rendered consistent with each other, at least to the extent that their relative conceptions of the psyche are not at odds with each other. Bringing these two approaches into something like harmony, without overlooking their incompatibilities, will be one of the tasks of the final chapter.

Furthermore, though Jung's treatment of adaptation focuses on typology, there is every reason to think that similar descriptions could be used for adaptation with respect to complexes (in Jung's sense of the term). For example, we might recognize that one's father complex is active and conscious at times in ways that are conducive to adaptation and the free "progression of libido," as when someone who is actually a father lives out his father complex consciously and appropriately. Yet we might also note that there are places where his father complex is unconsciously activated in ways which are not adaptive ("negative father complex") by, say, acting in a domineering and paternal or even paternalistic way toward coworkers. In a case like this, we would have to assume that an analogous cyclical pattern would apply, namely, that external adaptive problem entails the rendering conscious of the unconscious aspect of the complex which, in turn, allows the solution to the external problem, something which, in Jungian style, would contribute to the process of greater individuation. One does not need to look far in Jung to see just this situation in his clinical examples. Whether we speak of complexes, functions, or attitudinal directions (introversion and extraversion), the same pattern of treatment appears to obtain. Thus, what Jung describes in *On Psychic Energy* in purely typological terms should also be understood to apply directly to one's psychological relationship to specific complexes and consequently to the Jungian form of psychoanalytic treatment as a whole.

Adaptation in Clinical Practice

Central pieces of Langs' clinical theory are presaged in Jung's clinical theory. For example, decades before Langs' insistence on the "bi-personal field," Jung was arguing much the same point in *Psychology of the Transference* through alchemical images, such as the "bath" (Jung, 1946), something we also observed in chapter 1. This suggests that Jung had already in some measure moved beyond more monadic forms of thinking that Freud is sometimes criticized for, for example by relational psychoanalysts,[12] into a fully dyadic account of actual clinical processes. Indeed, even before *The Psychology of the Transference*, Jung developed ideas along the same axes in many of his clinical texts of the 1930s contained in volume 16 of the *Collected Works*. For example, in a 1935 lecture, "Principles of Practical Psychotherapy," Jung writes:

> A person is a psychic system which, when it affects another person, enters into a reciprocal reaction with another psychic system. This, perhaps the most modern, formulation of the psychotherapeutic relation between physician and patient is clearly very far removed from the original view that psychotherapy was a method which anybody could apply in stereotyped fashion in order to reach the desired results. (Jung, 1935: p. 1)

This "reciprocal reaction" suggests the adaptational principle that Langs also articulated, namely, that a primary source of adaptation is the therapeutic

---

12. Relational psychoanalysts have not, it seems, appreciated the extent to which Freud too was dyadic in his clinical theory, even if he was monadic in his theory of the psyche. Lothane has pertinent remarks here which would also apply in many ways to Jung (Lothane, 1997; Lothane, 2003).

relationship itself and that that adaptational relationship goes both ways, each member of the clinical dyad adapting to the other.[13]

However, beyond the parallels between Langs' and Jung's ideas, there is one piece where Jung goes a good deal beyond Langs: the importance of symbol for resolving adaptive conflicts. In many works, Jung develops his notion of the symbol and how the symbol "canalizes libido" (i.e., aids, through analogy, in re-directing psychic energy toward new and potentially fruitful places in one's life). According to Jung, symbols are not consciously or intentionally formed but are "always produced out of the unconscious by way of revelation or intuition" (Jung, 1948: para. 92). Jung believes that we are always and right from the start confronted with symbol formation in our patients, but these formations are typically unsuitable for adequate development—for the obvious reason that they represent the current, inadequate form of adaptation which includes the various ways that the flow of libido is dammed, and the person feels stuck. Hence, the given symbols, as a rule, must be analyzed and broken into their primitive parts, in order to restore something like a natural flow of energy. This aspect of analysis Jung considered to be "reductive," because it "reduces" the symbols to their historical and displaced or projected elements. However, according to Jung, as part of the teleology embedded in the human psyche as well as because of an innate excess of psychic energy, there is also a natural striving for a better energy gradient. Hence, Jung writes, once the natural flow of energy is restored, reductive analysis should end and symbol formation should "be reinforced in a synthetic direction until a more favorable gradient for the excess libido is found" (Jung, 1948: para. 94).

Jung sees such "synthetic direction" in the formation of symbols in religion and cultural development generally, as well as clinically in the dreams and fantasies of patients. Indeed, in principle the same symbols have both a reductive and synthetic meaning; the issue is often not whether there is a symbol to be interpreted synthetically or teleologically but whether it is the time for such a synthetic interpretation in the clinical process. It is of the nature of symbols—in contrast, for example, to concepts—that they are multivalent and thus one and the same symbol can in principle include both reductive and synthetic elements. If a man has an erotically charged dream of a female friend of the family, the dream certainly can indicate something of an erotic issue that requires a reductive analysis, but it can just as well (and in principle simultaneously) be an anima image, suggesting some definite movement toward individuation that has nothing specifically to do with exercising erotic interests. The material as well as the rhythm and movement of treatment are what usually give insight into which interpretive direction is more relevant at the time. Synthetic symbol formation is not only a description of

---

13. Lothane posits a similar relationship and a similar language in describing the clinical process between patient and analyst as when he discusses "reciprocal free association" in the analytic process (Lothane, 2010).

what the psyche does; it is also indicative specifically of its teleological orientation, something Jung developed in *Symbols of Transformation* (Jung, 1952) as well as some extensive passages in *Psychological Types* (Jung, 1923: para. 170–71).

We know from Jung's description that adaptation requires a change of attitude along the lines of the "functional types" as well as the "attitudinal types" (introversion and extraversion), such that our less developed sides are meant to come more to the fore and be developed. If adaptation is as central to the movements of the psyche toward individuation as Jung's description suggests, we would expect to find relevant and teleologically based symbols present in the patient's own material implying just this need, whether derived from dreams, language, fantasies, or transference experiences.

Returning to Bruce

I want now to return to the case of Bruce, in order to see what we can draw from his material with Jung's understanding of adaptation in mind. One would think that (1) if Jung's conception of adaptation is largely on target and (2) if Jung's view is potentially coherent with, rather than in contradiction to, Langs' conception of adaptation, as I have suggested earlier, we would be able to read from Bruce's material something of an illustration of Jung's ideas.

At this stage of Bruce's life, he was in a profession that demanded a good deal of intellectual rigor. Bruce, though intellectually gifted and having a robust thinking function, nonetheless had another side of him that was in some respects left latent through his profession, though it was much more alive at earlier stages of his life, namely, his feeling life. In fact, Bruce had at one time written poetry and loved art and images, giving the impression that an imaginative side of his personality deeply rooted in his feeling function was somehow frozen.

Some of the feeling issues, it would seem, were expressed from the beginning in Bruce's insistence on "cheap Jungian therapy." While this desire on his part might appear to be a purely practical consideration— just how it appeared to him—in practice wanting cheap therapy appeared to be simultaneously a symbol: a symbol of value or, more precisely, of devaluation of some kind, certainly of his own treatment and perhaps of his own psychic life as well as quite possibly a devaluation of me, his "cheap therapist." Since he was making a comfortable enough living to pay the fuller price for the therapy he was receiving, there was certainly more than just a practical situation at hand.

"Devaluations" of any kind will suggest to a Jungian an issue with feeling. Jung considers the feeling function what he would call a "rational function," in the sense that it corresponds to something in the world, namely, to values (Jung, 1923). In this respect, the feeling function is analogous to the thinking function: just as the thinking function relates to the nature of reality, feeling relates to what is experienced as valuable in reality. For example, when someone claims they have "strong feelings" about something, they are of course not simply speaking of their emotional or affective life; they are in essence saying that some question of significant value is at stake.

Now I emphasize Jung's description of the rationality of feeling because the language of "value" in English almost invariably has a subjective overtone it probably does not in Jung, thus inviting misunderstanding of Jung's point. In English-language thinking, it is typical for the term "value" to mean "something someone (potentially even arbitrarily) likes or prefers," thereby treating value as a placeholder for personal preferences. Yet the philosophical world in which Jung worked, including some philosophers he at times refers to (like Friedrich Nietzsche and Max Scheler) as a rule did *not* take the term "value" (*der Wert*) to mean some surrogate for something that is really "nothing but" a projection of personal desire. At this point in German-language philosophy, social science, and cultural theory, that is to say in the intellectual milieu in which Jung worked, value was generally understood to be a genuine, non-material and typically *felt* quality of reality (i.e., to be a real and experienced part of the furniture of the world, not simply a projection of individual preference [see, e.g., Scheler, 1973; White, forthcoming]).[14] Most of the German-language value philosophers of the time, whether phenomenological, neo-Kantian, or other, took beauty to be the prototypical case of value: beauty is something which does not arise from our mere subjective preferences but rather is experienced as something which strikes us with its own force, something which—as we put it in chapter 2—bursts through our encrusted subjectivity, demanding, as it were, that we appreciate something precious and worthy in itself quite beyond our preferences. Generalizing from the relatively clear example of beauty, we should understand that when Jung speaks of "value," he does not speak simply of subjective preference but rather of something that he believes is given directly in the world of our experience as an actual quality or attribute of things and which is independent of our desires, preferences, and so forth. This is what phenomenologists would call the "intentionality" of feeling, distinguishing thereby the feeling per se from the value to which it has reference: the *feeling* is internal to the psyche, but the *value quality being felt* is in the world, just as a cognition might be a psychic reality, but the object cognized is in the world (Scheler, 1973; Scheler, 1973a).

---

14. Contrast, for example, Sharp (1987) who simply takes for granted that any reference to value must be subjective. Quenk and Quenk try harder to understand the "rationality" of the feeling function by interpreting the function as a value judgment (1982). Yet here again, the excluded possibility (which appears to be Jung's intent), namely, *that one can feel value qualities in the world*, is never entertained, though a careful reading and thinking through of his definition of value feeling *Psychological Types*, suggests my interpretation. This exclusion of my interpretation is born more, I believe, of the impact of positivism and empiricism on English-language culture than of being an adequate reading of Jung.

It is in fact for this reason that the analogy Jung makes between think-ing and feeling, such that thinking and feeling are both "rational" functions, makes sense: they both treat of what is there in the world, one concerning the *nature* of reality (thinking), the other concerning its *value* (feeling).[15] While I realize such an approach is likely to be found both confusing in a highly materialist culture as well as potentially implausible, due at least in some measure to the strongly empiricist orientation of both academic and mental health cultures in the English-speaking world, it is important at the least that we recognize the likelihood of this interpretation of Jung. Jung lived in a world and posited an overall theory which was in part reacting against the empiricism and materialism of his time. His implicit understanding of value was one of the places where this reaction becomes especially manifest.

Assuming, then, this picture of a phenomenological link between the feeling function and value, we can perhaps shed some light Bruce's case. Given Bruce's own statement about the development of his thinking and rationality, given his stilted imagination and feeling life, and further given his devaluing of himself and his treatment by wanting "cheap therapy," already from the beginning there was more than a hint in the derivative material that a part of Bruce's one-sidedness and adaptive problems were bound up with a largely unconscious relationship to his feeling function. As a highly cultivated man, Bruce was clearly in contact with value as an intellectual phenomenon; he could *see* and *understand* value. The issue, one might speculate, was: could he *feel* values? That is to say, was his feeling function alive and awakened enough to be emotionally impacted by the values he saw, and could such experiences help resolve the neurotic issues which brought him into treatment? His original attitude toward his "cheap therapy" was already a derivative communication that his adaptive contexts would coagulate around issues of feeling and value, something which he himself also brought up incidentally in the opening session. Read along the lines of Langs' Type Two derivative, Bruce unconsciously devalued the therapeutic process as well as his therapist, something I took as a call both to bring feeling life and a sense for value into the consulting room, compensating in our process where Bruce could not yet do so individually.

Following Jung's description of an intensification of affect around adaptive issues, we can see a few places in the material which indicate Bruce's difficulties with his own feeling function. For example, in the last chapter, I emphasized communication issues and how Bruce's derivatives indicated psychic conflict around the tape recorder being the room. We recall that

---

15. This is, of course, a cursory treatment of a thorny problem, but it would take us too far afield to develop it in detail. Let it at least be stated that the philosophical world in which Jung worked did not think that five physical senses to be the only accesses to the world, as is typical in the English-speaking world imbued as it is with positivistic theory, but also took the psychic functions of thinking and feeling as directly and intuitively related to the world. In this respect, Jung parallels a good deal of the work of the early phenomenologists. Concerning especially the feeling of value qualities, chapter 1 of Scheler (1973) and Scheler (1973a) are most *a propos*.

Bruce made his proclamation into the tape recorder about not being homosexual with a good deal of humor but also with a powerful affective charge. Indeed, after he had made his pronouncement into the tape recorder, he told me he had had no homosexual experience; when I asked about homosexual feelings, he answered ambivalently that he "didn't really" have any. We were then to discover some thirty sessions later that Bruce had had some homosexual experience, that it had been deeply conflictual for him, and that it was a set of experiences, memories, and feelings toward which he was substantially closed off. We recall also that one of the disturbing experiences in the session was the cavalier, intellectualized way he spoke about what was clearly a deeply felt violation. Only when he had to speak of his relationship with his male teacher and the reaction of the retired child psychologist did he intimate that he had had homosexual experiences at all, let alone any that felt violating or emotionally painful. Standard defenses against feelings around valuable aspects of personality, such as sexuality, were clearly at work, above all intellectualization—which emphasizes thinking at the expense of feeling—and a specific form of denial—the denial bound up with the value of an experience, represented in his cavalier attitude toward himself—rendering some substantial aspect of Bruce's feeling function closed off and stuck. For this reason, we can read the derivatives around the tape recorder as *both* suggesting an unconscious conflict about the tape recorder *and* indicative of a long-term issue with his own feeling function. We can also recognize in them a fear that I will violate his feeling and his sense of his own value, just as the psychologist did—a Type Two derivative reading of the situation.

Furthermore, one reason Bruce was closed off to this aspect of his psychological life was that the person to whom he had originally entrusted the information, his former child psychologist, had acted in a way that indicated to Bruce that this painful chapter of his life and the feeling and value aspects of it were "too hot for anyone to handle," that something in the feeling and value content of this experience required it be tucked away in the unconscious and not again brought to light. If he couldn't even trust the psychologist to manage this part of Bruce's psychological life without brutalizing him, to whom was he to entrust it? That being the case, we can assume that one adaptive task he needed to deal with was that some substantial part of his feeling life around sexuality was closed off, something confirmed by the difficulties he had speaking about these issues. I note in passing that a broader analysis of his material confirmed these points, including conflicts associated with his two previous marriages (he was on his third).

Furthermore, as he spoke about the experiences of his adolescent relationship with his teacher and the later betrayal by the child psychologist, I seemed to feel the emotional devastation that Bruce could not: I felt not only my own pain and empathy but some of his pain and anguish that he could not seem to carry, as if he did not have the psychic resources to endure the specific feeling quality of this pain or of the experience of the violation of the values that had been associated with his budding adolescent sexuality. Indeed, the most challenging part of the session for me was hearing him make fun of his wounded self, with cavalier and sarcastic language, as if his younger, more emotional self was foolish and stupid precisely for feeling the pain in a way we would quite expect from an adolescent boy. It was as if Bruce persecuted the very feeling life of the boy he was, its character and quality.

The changes in Bruce's mode of communication that occurred after we removed the recorder buttressed this point. Bruce lost a good deal of his stiffness, to be sure, but more importantly he not only began to allow himself to feel and process his own pain, but purposely decided to take the couch for a dozen or so sessions, with the aim of getting more in touch with his feeling life. Bruce succeeded in communicating with his feeling life in many ways from that point on, recalling, for example, early life events previously forgotten, some of them profoundly significant for the man he had become. Before treatment ended, Bruce could communicate with some of his own deep feelings and the correlating violations of his own self-value and disappointments especially in his mother as real parts of himself, not by taking the "side" of a persecutory thinking function against his feeling function. Among these deeper experiences were repressed feelings about maternal failures, permitting himself both negative feelings toward and negative evaluations of his mother, which he could not admit at first in treatment.

It is important to notice that many of the same symbols and images that we examined in the last chapter and interpreted as primarily pertaining to the external adaptive context alone, such as the cost of therapy and the impact of the tape recorder in the room, *also* derivatively expressed symbols of the inner adaptive context and the inner adaptation that Bruce had to make. That there was a communicative breakdown going on in our work was clear and that that breakdown was expressed through "cheap therapy" (i.e., therapy reduced in quality through the use of a tape recorder as an unconscious defense against communication). But it should also be clear that there was a prior communicative breakdown enacted in Bruce's own soul when he consciously and unconsciously shut down his inner feeling and imaginative life in favor of the highly rationalistic one. On the surface, this freed Bruce from the struggles of having to feel the pain associated with his violated sexual life and with evaluations he would have to make accordingly, like admitting that he and his sexuality had been deeply violated, that his violation was in some way so bad that his former psychologist couldn't handle it without experiencing it as seductive, and that he had not gained much by way of parental protection from this situation due, among other things, to his mother's poor choices in partners, who also did not do much to initiate Bruce into manhood. These repressed and at times barely remembered struggles reoccurred when he first came to therapy and found that his conscious, thinking life began to relate to his unconscious feeling life and imagination, something that must have felt to him very much like the "nosy supervisor" we discussed in the last chapter (read as a Type One derivative), refusing to mind its own business, something he also originally felt toward me (Type Two derivative). Bruce defended against his feeling life by keeping an external "recorder" in the room—a substitute for an internal recording and recalling of his own feeling life. And only when we banished the substitute recorder from the room would his own inner recorder, with its memories of painful experiences and feelings, communicate first with himself and then with me.

The strength of Langs' approach, which was essential to my work with Bruce, was that it could highlight the external adaptive context and aid me in the work of correcting a frame that was not conducive to the symbolizing field needed for us to get to the genuinely deeper, emotional work and healing Bruce needed. Jung's understanding of adaptation, however, supplemented that work by adding an inner dimension of adaptation that Langs' work could never quite articulate, namely, that in order to resolve the outer adaptive problem—in Bruce's case, the limits to psychological insight and development imposed by the tape recorder being in the room— we simultaneously need to resolve the inner adaptive context, in this case restoring the inner communication between Bruce's conscious, thinking form of adaptation and his unconscious, underused feeling kind of adaptation. Only when the process finally "came to a head," when Bruce had to make a choice *either* to remain locked in a thinking-based and intellectualized communicative system, intrapsychically and interpersonally, *or* banish the tape recorder and be willing to live his feeling life in some measure, along with its painful memories, could he finally marshal sufficient psychic energy to make the necessary move.

The relevant adaptive context was therefore not exactly within or without but rather where the outer and the inner mirrored each other. It was when the intrapsychic communicative breakdown and the interpersonal communicative breakdown in some sense reflected each other that finally enough dammed-up psychic energy and frustrating affect could emerge for Bruce to put both his external defense (tape recorder) and internal defenses (defenses against feeling) away. This example should intimate to us that there is something in the insights of both Langs and Jung that supplement each other when it comes to adaptive problems.

Now this use of derivative communication on my part for validating typology is not something which is typically discussed in Jungian literature. The reason for that is that the typical approach to typology is through clinical observation (or possibly self-tests) and that is often deemed sufficient to know someone's typology. While it might be true that in some cases observation is sufficient, as mentioned earlier in this chapter, issues of typology are perhaps more subtle than they seem. For example, a person's developed persona might emphasize a specific typological category but outside of professional or social contexts, that same person might act from a quite different, dominating typology. Consequently, even if it were true that clinical observation is usually sufficient for understanding the typology of one's patient—something that appears questionable in at least some cases to this clinician—there is still benefit from recognizing that the unconscious communications on the part of the patient may verify which specific functional directions of the patient are in need of therapeutic care.

Clarifying Adaptation in Jung

The analysis and example in this chapter highlight the dynamic sense of adaptation in Jung, a meaning of adaptation which refers to a basic dynamism in the psyche, which we also contrasted with a different and substantially more common meaning of adaptation in Jung, the sense of being "collectively minded." The latter is a more or less negative sense of adaptation and is often the one referred to by Jungian authors, who appear not to have noticed the other more positive meaning of adaptation in Jung.

A case in point is Dieckmann's fine book on analytic practice (Dieckmann, 1991). In a chapter on working with various age groups, Dieckmann offers some criticisms of Jolande Jacobi, Michael Fordham, and others, who appear to view adaptation as an essential part of the individuation process. Dieckmann points out that "Jacobi goes far beyond Jung's definition of the concept [of individuation] which opposed individuation to the collective psyche and the processes of adaptation" (Dieckmann, 1991: p. 92). Dieckmann continues in the same vein throughout the chapter, trying to offer greater subtlety to how adaptation and individuation might be related, since they are, in practice, opposed to each other.

Without entering into the details of these discussions, we may at least say that Dieckmann is certainly correct in thinking that one of the meanings of "adaptation" in Jung is typically contrary to individuation and that that meaning is certainly the one that Dieckmann highlights, namely, being collectively minded and too defined by collective mores and attitudes. Furthermore, it is easy to find passages in Jung which express points cognate to those made by Dieckmann. For example, in one of his clinical essays, Jung highlights that psychoneuroses can be divided into two main groups,

> the one comprising collective people with underdeveloped individuality, the other individualists with atrophied collective adaptation. The therapeutic attitude differs accordingly, for it is abundantly clear that a neurotic individualist can only be cured by recognizing the collective man in himself—hence the need for a collective adaptation. It is therefore right to bring him down to collective truth. On the other hand, psychotherapists familiar with the collectively adapted person who has everything and does everything that could reasonably be required as a guarantee of health, but yet is ill. It would be a bad mistake, which is nevertheless very often committed, to normalize such a person and try to bring him down to the collective level. (Jung, 1935: p. 7)

The latter part of this passage clearly uses "adaptation" in the collective sense highlighted above. Similarly, Jung's schematic writing entitled "Adaptation, Individuation, Collectivity" (Jung, 1977) also treats adaptation as a kind of opposite to individuation, even to the point of posing the adapted person as inherently collectivist and contrasting such a person to one truly seeking individuation as being unadapted to the collective.

At the same time, this analysis illustrates the sharp differences between adaptation in this collective sense and adaptation in the dynamic sense. Certainly, if one means by "adaptation" the collective sense of the term, it is typically not conducive to individuation—though earlier in the quoted passage we see that Jung recognizes that some people actually need to become more collectively minded, suggesting the issue is not as cut and dried as Dieckmann thinks. Yet even if we were to assume Dieckmann's analysis to be correct, he would still have to account for the very different sense of adaptation that Jung develops in *On Psychic Energy*, which has no inherent connection to being collectively minded and which clearly, both conceptually and descriptively, works in the direction of individuation by evoking both the unconscious compensatory function of the psyche and sufficient conscious affect to demand of the person in question that they develop underdeveloped functions of the psyche. Rather than being inimical to individuation, this sense of adaptation describes a dynamic dimension of the psyche, whereby one expands one's psychic energies and resources by making relatively unconscious orientations and attitudes more conscious and more functional. Adaptation in the full dynamic sense of the term is a process directed by the Self and conducive to individuation because it forces a redirecting and, ultimately, the enhancement and differentiation of conscious psychic energy.

Conclusion

Approaching adaptation from Jung's dynamic sense of the term reveals important aspects of the adaptive process, including elements which Langs either leaves out or perhaps cannot countenance given his theoretical assumptions. Jung's treatment of adaptation in *On Psychic Energy*, though somewhat cursory from the standpoint of volume, goes a good way toward treating adaptation as a long-term process, one clearly bound up with the basic teleology of the psyche and latter's goal of individuation or wholeness. Further, in certain respects, Jung's treatment offers a more properly psychological treatment of adaptation than Langs, in that he recognizes adaptation as a psychological process, rather than exclusively a psychological reaction to an external adaptive stimulus. In certain ways, in fact, Langs' and Jung's treatments of adaptation are different enough that it might seem one cannot bring them into something like a harmony, at least sufficient to find them both useful clinically.

However, as the example of Bruce showed, not only can each of these approaches to adaptation be useful in a given clinical situation; at times, the same clinical material appears useful for each approach. Consequently, there are grounds for thinking not only that each of these approaches can in principle be used together but that the same material can illuminate each approach, even though each approach is in some sense asking different questions and surveying different aspects of psychic development and healing for the patient. This fact suggests that Langs' and Jung's approach to adaptation are less two different conceptualizations of the same process than highlighting two different elements of the adaptive process in general.

In the next and final chapter, we will attempt to bring these two approaches to something of a unity and try to generate some principles for understanding adaptive issues in the clinical setting. In one respect, this will be a very Langsian approach because of its focus on technical principles, though the development of Jungian ideas in this chapter will modify how we understand Langs' insights. We will have to begin with some discussion, however, of a general resistance to treating of issues of technique in the Jungian community.

CHAPTER 5

Adaptation and Clinical Technique

Introduction

The Jungian tradition in general—though not every specific subtradition within it—speaks little of clinical technique, especially as compared to the many articles and books in the Freudian tradition on technique, beginning already with some of Freud's classic essays. In fact, one can get the impression from some respected sources in the Jungian literature not only that there is no specifically Jungian clinical technique but that any emphasis or perhaps even any discussions of technique should be avoided. Consequently, before we attempt to establish some clinical precepts, it is incumbent that we consider some of the objections to treatments of clinical technique in analytical psychology. Both the nature of the dispute as well as the preliminary considerations offered in response may be of interest not only to Jungians but to readers outside the Jungian tradition as well.

Considerations of clinical technique have produced a certain amount of controversy in analytical psychology, something we can see perhaps best through the eyes of the "Zürich" versus the "London" traditions. On the one hand, the classically trained Gerhard Adler, representing the Zürich approach (though writing about it while living in England), writes that the:

> most important limitation [on discussions of clinical technique] is due to the fact that one of the main differences between Analytical Psychology and other schools lies in the undogmatic approach of Analytical Psychology to each individual case. The basic presupposition from which Analytical Psychology starts is that each patient has his own and "personal" psychology necessitating an approach which changes with each individual case. . . . Such a conception must obviously involve a considerable limitation on general technique, since the whole point of a technique is to provide certain universally applicable rules. (Adler, n.d.: p. 22)

In contrast to Adler—and to some extent intentionally so—the London School, which developed around the work of Michael Fordham and in which there is a good deal more intermingling of Freudian and Jungian thinking, focused much of its attention on clinical technique. For example, authors of this school published an entire volume entitled *Technique in Jungian Analysis*, dedicated to approaches to working with the transference and countertransference (Fordham et al., 1974). Indeed, in his substantial book review of Robert Langs' volumes on technique entitled *The Therapeutic Interaction*, Fordham bemoaned the lack of consideration of technique in the Jungian tradition and considered Langs' work something of an ideal for how he wished analytical psychologists would work (Fordham, 1978). Fordham, in contrast to Adler, appears to have no aversion to treating clinical technique. However, Fordham and those associated with him also appear to be a minority in this regard among analytical psychologists. The general scarcity of other books originally in English either on some aspect of clinical technique or collecting articles on clinical technique in analytical psychology since Fordham's 1974 collection highlights this issue.[1]

The earlier quotation from Adler aptly expresses one side of the controversy, while also indicating some of the anxieties which seem to provoke his stated reaction. One motivation for this reaction, as we suggested in this book's introduction, is a certain assumption about the meaning of individuation. The term "individuation" appears to have two somewhat diverse meanings in Jungian thought, meanings which are not typically or adequately differentiated in Jungian literature. On the one hand, individuation refers to the general teleology and movement of the psyche toward wholeness, the term "individuation" being derived from the Latin *individuum*, meaning "undivided unity." On the other hand, individuation has always also had the connotation (including in Jung's work) of indicating a movement toward being differentiated from unconscious collectives. While both of these meanings are present in much of the Jungian tradition, they are neither the same in meaning nor in extension, for reasons already outlined in the introduction to this volume.

It does not take much consideration to recognize that this second sense of "individuation" is also at the root of some of the confusions in the Jungian literature concerning adaptation. For what we termed the "collective sense" of adaptation in the last chapter is functionally opposite of and correlative to "individuation" in the second sense just outlined, since "adaptation" in the collective sense consists in an unconscious identification with the collective, rather than achieving differentiation from it (individuation in the second sense). It is no doubt largely for this reason that adaptation is usually considered a negative for Jung and Jungians because it is assumed that adaptation implies the opposite of individuation. While we cannot enter into this set of conceptual problems in detail at this point (though these and previous comments throughout this study offer some clarification), it is evident for

---

1. A recent and refreshing exception to this rule is Mark Winborn's fine book on interpretation, entitled *Interpretation in Jungian Analysis* (Winborn, 2019). Hans Dieckmann's book on technique was translated into English from German in the 1990s, but nothing similar has been written in English.

our purposes both that (1) the proper sense of individuation is the first sense mentioned since it is the universal sense attributed to the psyche, whereas the second sense is not universal, in that some people's process toward wholeness requires they become somewhat more collective ("consciously communal" would be a better term)—thus, the second meaning of "individuation" must be a derivative and secondary meaning of the term—and (2) we will be concerned here with adaptation in the dynamic rather than the collective sense, just as we were in the previous chapter, since this is the sense that is actually conducive to individuation in the proper (first) sense of the term.

A second anxiety implied in Adler's quotation is that the development of universal principles of technique in some measure contradicts the "undogmatic approach of Analytical Psychology." The implication of this passage appears to be that if one articulates general precepts of technique, then one by some inner necessity must become "dogmatic." This assumption on Adler's part is evidently a purposeful and rhetorical exaggeration, utilized to highlight a point. "Dogmatism" in its usual sense is less a term describing propositions or practices (such as technique) than a term highlighting the way in which those propositions or practices are held or utilized by a given person. One is "dogmatic" not because one admits general principles but because one holds to them in a way which is too rigid, either by interpreting them too literally and formulaically or by treating them as so exclusive that one refuses to entertain possible exceptions to them. Thus, while Adler raises a potentially important point here, namely, that principles of technique should not be held dogmatically but should rather be conceived of as somewhat flexible generalities, he appears to overstate his case by attributing the problem of dogmatism to the very formulation of technique, rather than to a lack of flexibility in its application by a given person and in a given case.

Finally, Adler seems to suggest that any formulation of general principles of technique amounts to an implicit violation of the individual and personal psychology of the patient. Once again, we appear to have a rhetorical exaggeration in order to make a point. To suggest that any clinical stance which includes general principles of technique violates individual psychology frankly borders on the bizarre. For one, taken literally, it would suggest that any tradition which considers general principles of technique important is, just by virtue of that, indifferent to the demands of individual and personal psychology, as if, say, classical Freudian psychoanalysts don't care about individual psychology insofar as they are concerned with general principles technique—an implausible idea to say the least. Quite the contrary, it is important for any practicing depth psychological practitioner to have at least some principles for the use of practical technique, without which one would be reinventing the wheel each time one sees a patient and without which one cannot really improve on one's practice because, rather than developing actual technical habits which can in turn be improved upon, one eschews general habits all together in the name of some supposed radical individuality on the part of the patient. Indeed, all general knowledge of technique plus specific principles associated with specific diagnoses would have to be taken as a violation of the patient, were we to take Adler's point literally, since he suggests that general principles just by virtue of being general violate individual psychology. Rather than walking down the path of such a *reductio ad absurdum*, one that is unintelligible except in terms of extreme rhetorical exaggeration, the valuable point we need to take from Adler is that one needs to be careful *in the application* of general principles and not apply them in a mechanical, universalistic, or ruthless way, without individual nuance. Though an excellent point, it appears to be overstated and to some extent misdirected in this passage.

In contrast to Adler's formulations here, it should be noted that, as much as one should appreciate the individual psychology of each patient, it is equally important to recognize the value of one's accumulated knowledge of human nature in general as well as broad specifics (e.g., experiences of specific psychopathologies), as important factors for one's work with patients as well. Though there are certainly valuable points to be drawn from his view, Adler's rhetorical exaggerations express an enantiadromic leap from one extreme—the highlighted potential dangers of an overemphasis on technique and generalities—to the opposite extreme of more or less avoiding the formulation of clinical principles and generalities entirely, due to an alleged danger to analytic practice embedded in the very formulation of technique itself and by misattributing dogmatism and poor technique to the formulation of technique itself rather than the person wielding it. What Adler underlines quite well is that there is an approach to technical considerations that divorces the latter from the actual concerns for the patient, something which certainly should be avoided. However, it seems to follow from these points only that one should be careful about how one formulates and understands principles of clinical technique, not that one should avoid them as if they are inherent dangers.

Given the intensity of the controversy over technique in the Jungian world, perhaps some general points about technique are merited. As is often the case in such disputes, there are valid points to each side and it behooves us to take each side into account—especially the values that each side represents, if not always the literal statements expressed.

What Is and What Is the Value of Clinical Technique?

Notions of "technique," "analytic technique," "clinical technique," and the like are central to analytic practice. By "technique" we mean any activity undertaken by the practitioner of a specific discipline or social practice, because it is conducive to the end, purpose, or goal of that discipline or practice. I offer this rough and ready definition in a way that is broad enough to include basically any purposeful activity within a general practice of any kind, whether the way an offensive lineman uses his body, the way the violinist holds the bow during a certain solo passage, the manner in which the organic gardener mixes the compost, or the manner in which a psychotherapist offers an interpretation to a patient's dream. The definition is also narrow enough to reduce what counts as "technical" exclusively to those practices which are also *intended to be such* by the practitioner. By way of example, the "frame" of therapy is not a technique, but how a therapist uses the frame for the purposes of therapy is (or at least can be) a technique. The fee for therapy is not a technique per se; the manner in which the fee is arranged, the fee agreement is formulated, the policies designed with a potentially therapeutic purpose, along with paying attention to how all these factors might appear in patient material are all examples of technique or at least of practices which can evaluated from the standpoint of technique. While Jungians at times speak loosely, say, of active imagination as "a technique," strictly speaking it is only a technique when, insofar, and in the manner that it is used to further the goal of therapy or analysis (or some other goal), not when it is considered independently of some goal. The crucial point to be drawn from this is that anything worthy of the name "technique" must be understood in the context of the social practice in which it is being utilized and in terms of its conscious purpose.

Often, for pedagogical purposes, we discuss therapeutic techniques outside of their actual use and context. For example, one might consider what makes a "good interpretation" by looking at the formulation of an interpretation, its tone, its style, and so forth. Such an approach can be fruitful and may permit a student of the analytic craft to focus their mind on formal elements and characteristics of an interpretation. However, as is always the case with discussions of technique—clinical, psychological, or otherwise— the point is not to assume that such formal characteristics are sufficient either for understanding or for mastering the technique in question. For the purposes of examining what one is doing, one might evaluate an interpretation outside of its function in a particular therapeutic process; yet the interpretation cannot be evaluated comprehensively based solely on those formal characteristics, precisely because it must ultimately be understood in terms of the goals of the specific practice. If I tell someone that they have offered a "good interpretation" to the patient, I am not simply saying that the interpretation fits all the formal requirements that make something a well-formulated interpretation; I also mean it was *effective*, actually or potentially, because it was conducive either to the near objectives of the session or perhaps to the more distant goals of the process as a whole.

In fact, in general we can say that the value of any technique is measured in (at least) a two-fold way: (1) as an example of good craftsmanship and (2) as a piece of a larger, purposeful process. I can, for example, give a well-crafted interpretation but do it at a time in a session where active listening rather than interpretation is called for. The evaluation of a technique is always two-fold: as a self-standing example of the craft (e.g., "is it a well-crafted intervention?") and from the standpoint of the therapeutic process (e.g., "is this productive or likely to be productive of the patient's healing?"). In this respect, technique in therapy is just like technique in all practical disciplines. A linebacker may make an excellent block but block the wrong person or at the wrong time, thus throwing off the process, in this case a football play, as a whole. The craft is there but the sense for the process is not. And so on with most kinds of technique.

In the Jungian tradition, emphasis tends to be given (1) to the value of the overall process and (2) to the way healing has to do with the relationship between analyst and analysand. These points should be accepted as valid, to be sure, and there is no substitute for the healing nature of the relationship or the quality of the analyst. Indeed, this latter point in well-established beyond the confines of analytic forms of therapy (e.g., in the therapeutic research of Wampold, which shows more or less definitively that the primary effectiveness in psychotherapy derives from two variables: (1) the working alliance and (2) the quality of the therapist [Wampold, 2001; Wampold, 2010]). In analytic traditions, these two factors have in fact generally been emphasized, the working alliance being formulated decades ago by Ralph Greenson, the quality of the therapist supposedly guaranteed by the trainee themselves having been analyzed. Yet there is perhaps less an emphasis on the craft and technical aspect of analysis in the Jungian world than there might be. The reasons for this lack of emphasis, however, need to be brought into focus.

We mentioned earlier that a technique is typically a part of a *social practice*. By calling it "social," we are referring to it two-dimensionally (i.e., both as a practice of a social group but also as a practice born of tradition). Though a contemporary analyst might easily see the significance of the first—after all, one learns analysis from others so there is a clear social component in the first sense—it might not be equally obvious that therefore it is also a practice with a tradition and, furthermore, that the fact it has a tradition matters for the practice. In our time, people frequently think of traditions to be largely unconscious practices which are by definition burdensome or outdated and thus turn to new sources for their understanding of techniques (in any discipline). However, the risk of such an approach is that something experienced as "burdensome" or "outdated" may not in fact be obsolete, but simply such that one doesn't recognize the original reasons and motives behind it, such as what problem it was designed to solve; hence it may not be that the technique is outdated but that its context has become lost or forgotten.

The reason this is important is that the formulation of good technique is invariably a function of the fact that it has been practiced by a number of people and over a substantial period of time, by people who can compare notes, share proprietary information, who can and do debate over what counts as good technique and why, and so forth—it is engendered and fine-tuned through tradition. Once technique is formulated, it tends to be treated in abstraction from the sets of experiences which engendered it. Thus, for example, one could teach a budding analyst some of the "rules" of dream interpretation without necessarily cluing the neophyte in to the experiences and insights worked through in the analytic tradition which engendered those rules of interpretation. Because of the abstraction which comes with the formulation of technical rules, especially in analytic education, such that rules may be taught without also explaining and articulating the experiences which engendered them—unfortunately an all-too-common occurrence in all forms of education—it is always possible and perhaps even likely that many a practitioner will be aware of the rule but not the background experiences, experiences which amount to the empirical sources and justifications for the technical rules. The candidate practitioner will thus be left to wonder about why a technical rule, precept, or formulation was articulated in the first place or possibly in the end just reject it because of ignorance of the experiences in the tradition which also justify the rule. Such approaches will often result in the loss of the tradition as an important epistemological guide in what counts as good practice.

When some technical rule has existed over many generations of practitioners, there typically are massive amounts of concrete empirical experience lying behind the techniques. In cases like this, it is not sufficient, in this writer's opinion, simply to reject or ignore such practices; rather, one must explore and understand why the technical procedures were formulated, what problems they were intended to solve, and approach those techniques with an open, even if critical, mind. As with any living tradition, one can deviate from it, but it is important that one know both what one is deviating from and why one is doing so, lest one's individual experiences be given greater weight than the weight of a well worked-through tradition and, in the case of analytic practice, its substantial body of literary output.

These points may help to highlight some of the Jungian controversy concerning technique. It may be that Adler's concern was born of the fact that the accumulated wisdom of a tradition, such as psychoanalysis, can become formulated in petrified propositions formulated or taught in abstraction from the experiences and purposes for which they were originally engendered. The abstracted character of technical rules, especially when they are being taught as generalizations in the midst of analytic training, could in principle produce analysts who are technically proficient, in the sense that they understand the craft, but lack good clinical sensibilities about the art and the process which set the context of the technique. The former are rules and guidelines of the craft, but the craft itself is always part of an art, an art much more based on experience, observation, and hit-and-miss attempts, than the abstracted technical rules in themselves might suggest. Like any art, being good at analysis requires consistent experience, reflection, intuition, insight, and, above all, what the ancient philosophers called *phronesis*, a type of prudence whereby one understands and has the feel for the moment when the technique is to be used. It is certainly possible to focus on technique at the expense of the more important elements of analytic process born of relationship, especially since the latter generally includes a good deal more anxiety for the analyst or analyst-trainee than issues of technique produce.

Yet, on the other side of the issue, we should note that learning the craft is part of the art, an art which like nearly any long-practiced art includes accumulated wisdom, much of which is formulated as technique and in technical terms. Both the art itself and the typical manner of analytic education highlight the importance of these points. Typically, Jungian and Freudian analysts are trained not in a purely academic fashion but rather in the manner of a medieval guild, in a relationship of "apprentice" (candidate) to "master craftsman" (analyst). One introjects the art of analysis by watching one's own analyst at work as well as by experiencing various supervising analysts who monitor cases and guide students working with case material, with their research, and with their practices. Though this introjection should never be a mere imitation, there is some measure of imitation that is usually part of the process, until one learns how to "make the technique one's own." This is in fact typical to any craft, not only the analytic craft. Such experiences are at least meant to give a sense for both the art and the craft, and the approach succeeds when it does both. Indeed, there would hardly be reason for independent analytic training institutes if analysis could be taught simply as a craft; it is because it is an art, and an art that is not purely obtained through academic knowledge, that one needs an independent institute, comprised of capable practitioners of the art, and that one learns in a guild model which confers knowledge through observation, imitation, and practice. It is precisely because the craft can only be measured within the practice of an art best taught on the guild model that independent institutes are needed.[2]

From these admittedly schematic discussions concerning technique and associated issues, we can perhaps posit the following:

1. Technical considerations are not to be avoided in discussions of analytic practice, yet technical considerations should be understood as only a part of a larger therapeutic art and process and not as either ends in themselves or to consist in the entirety or even the most important part of the therapeutic art.[3]
2. Technical principles should be formulated in such a way that the individual psychologies of both analyst and patient can be acknowledged and accounted for, since only within the context of the working alliance can we determine what concretely is adequate from a technical

---

2. Medieval philosophers would have called this guild style of education a kind of "connatural" knowledge (i.e., something which is gained by first imitating and then by introjecting the work of masters and, over time, turning the principles internalized into one's own unique style).
3. In fact, Gill (1984) suggests that Langs does just that, namely, reduce the entire relationship between patient and therapist to technique.

standpoint—indeed, ideally, technical practices should be expressions of the working alliance.

3. However, technical considerations are a substantial part of the craft of analysis and bound up significantly with the tradition of depth psychology and with a model of training and research closely associated with the "craft guild." While technique is no substitute for the quality of the therapist or the working alliance, it nonetheless is an important aspect of analytic training and of therapeutic work itself and requires its own set of principles.

Though these points by no means exhaust the questions that would need to be answered for understanding the nature and value of psychoanalytic clinical technique, it is hoped that they treat the controversy within analytical psychology sufficiently for the reader to recognize the relative importance of any discussion of adaptation and technique. While we by no means wish to suggest that technique has a priority over either the individual psychology of the patient or the therapeutic relationship or working alliance (*pace* Adler), we nonetheless believe that reflection on technique and its proper usage, keeping in mind the priority of both working alliance and of individual depth and sophistication on the part of the analyst, is potentially conducive to making the analytical relationship more effective. Consequently, drawing some technical conclusions from our examination of Langs and Jung on adaptation should be of some value.

What Langs and Jung Share

Adaptation clearly plays an important role in both Langs' and Jung's clinical theories and their respective understandings of the psyche and its nature. Yet, as we have seen, their emphases are much different. Langs' understanding of both psyche and clinical practice hinges much more on a conception of adaptation than Jung, for whom adaptation (always understood in the dynamic sense) is a description of one of the basic movements of the psyche but hardly exhausts his conception of the psyche or could count as an entire "paradigm" of analysis. This difference, as we shall see, is not only a difference of emphasis but one of general orientation and of focus. The insight into the kind of priority adaptive issues has for understanding unconscious material appears to have so impressed Langs that, in certain respects, he dedicated the rest of his publishing life to working out its implications. By the end of his life, he had modified most of psychoanalytic theory to accommodate the range of insights he had concerning adaptation, basically organizing all of his theorizing around it: hence "the adaptive paradigm." Jung, in contrast, speaks explicitly of adaptation in the dynamic sense in only a few passages of his major texts, though throughout his work, especially in his descriptions of working with "feeling-toned complexes," he evidently assumes his description of adaptation. Rather than focusing all his attention on adaptation and its implications, Jung's orientation, as we saw last chapter, was more phenomenological and hermeneutic than scientific and thus he tended to want to expand the range of materials used to understand the psyche, including studies of religion, mythology, alchemy, esoteric psychology, and so forth, rather than focus on one albeit vital variable in clinical practice. Consequently, our two authors have very different mental orientations, a difference which is highlighted in their writings in general as well as in their respective developments of adaptation. Nonetheless, with a little work, we should be able to link their two conceptions together, to the extent that they are compatible with each other. We shall first look at areas where they seem to converge, then areas where they might converge or more properly complement each other, and finally other places where they seem to differ decisively, paying attention to clinical implications in each case.

In the process, we will also have to engage critically with each author, both fine-tuning our understanding of each author as well as offering criticism where their conceptions appear to be inadequate.

Both Langs and Jung consider "adaptation" to be an essential dynamism or orientation of the psyche, rooted in its nature, and both suggest, therefore, that recognizing and understanding how that essential dynamism is working in any specific case is a necessary part of clinical work, especially when it comes to understanding unconscious processes and communications. While Jung does not underline this point with the force or repetition that Langs does, this is not because he does not consider adaptation a necessary constituent for understanding clinical process and unconscious communication, we would suggest. It is rather because Jung seems to take the process he describes in terms of adaptation so for granted—as did most of the early analytic thinkers, as we discussed in chapter 2—that he seems not to think it needs to be emphasized. This point is easily seen from the fact that Jung *defines* consciousness in terms of adaptation, as we saw in chapter 4, delineating the psychological types as modes of adaptation. Consequently, for Jung, to the extent that clinical work includes conscious functioning as well as recognizing unconscious material in aid of making it conscious—a fairly straightforward description of analytic work in its classical acceptation—it must include adaptive considerations.

This all suggests that two places where Langs and Jung converge clinically is that (1) adaptive considerations are intrinsic and essential to clinical work and that (2) recognizing unconscious communications in clinical material is both aided by and requires the analyst's consciousness of adaptive issues, problems, and contexts. No Jungian I am aware of has either isolated adaptation in its dynamic sense in Jung or suggested that it is this important for understanding clinical material, even though all Jungians are aware of the various descriptions and mechanisms connected to adaptation, such as the intensification of affect around unconscious material (complexes), typological challenges, and compensation. In other words, nothing in what is described here is likely to be new to Jungian practitioners other than the claim that the interpretive grid on which Jung founds these basic experiences and mechanisms is based on his understanding of adaptation. Most likely, the failure to recognize the adaptive orientation in Jung derives from Jung himself and his failure to differentiate adaptation in the dynamic sense and adaptation in the collective sense. Once that it is clarified, however, we can not only bring adaptive issues into focus but also have some grounds for bringing ideas from Langs into dialogue with those of Jung.

Consequently, we can further say that adaptive issues appear, in Langs and Jung, as important factors in all psychic conflict. For Langs, adaptive issues seem to be by far the primary (or perhaps even the exclusive) factor producing psychic conflict and for Jung, insofar as psychic conflict arises from not being able to marshal either sufficient or the appropriate form of energy for a flowing progression of libido or psychic energy, adaptation is also for him a primary (and perhaps the primary) factor in psychic conflict. Though Jung's complicated psychic world which includes archetypes, layers of collectivity, alchemical processes, and so forth does not permit us to say that adaptive issues are the only factor in psychic conflict, we can nonetheless say that they are always a part of the reason for psychic conflict. Thus, we can draw the clinical principle from this that, to the extent that our patients come to us due to their experiencing psychic conflict, our case formulations and how we understand both the conflicts and their solutions requires that we understand something of the adaptive problems that (at least in part) produce the conflict.[4] Indeed, for some patients, recognizing that adaptive issues and their concomitant conflicts are in some ways inherent to psychological life and its expansion—something that Jung definitely believes—is potentially a beneficial piece of knowledge, depending on the needs of the patient.

Third, hearkening back to the example in the introduction, an adaptive focus tends to highlight *motivations*, both conscious and unconscious, for psychic conflicts as well as for feelings such as anxiety or depression. While this point is clear in Langs, whose focus on adaptation underlines this point in countless ways, it is a point at least as important for a Jungian practitioner. For if adaptation in the dynamic sense essentially describes progression and regression of psychic energy, then every attempt at concrete adaptation and especially every attempt at managing maladaptive reactions based on the relative unconsciousness of any complex or any of the four functions, amounts to a manifestation of the teleology of the psyche (i.e., the call to a greater balance in conscious orientation and to wholeness). Adaptive issues in

---

4. "The psychological trouble in neurosis, and the neurosis itself, can be formulated as *an act of adaptation that has failed*," (Jung, 1955: italics in original).

essence force the psyche to confront unconscious factors that are in some sense meant to be conscious as part of the movement toward wholeness. Adaptation operationalizes teleology: it concretizes Jung's relatively abstract principle of teleology into a definite, concrete, and in principle quantitative form (in the sense of "quantity" developed in the previous chapter). This would suggest, from a technical point of view, that consciousness of adaptive issues is a concrete way of becoming conscious not only of motivational factors in psychic conflict but also of both the teleology of the psyche and the specific movements of the compensatory function of the unconscious.

Thus, though there is a point of convergence between Langs and Jung, the situation is somewhat more complex than can be developed here in detail. For one, Langs clearly believes adaptive issues and especially externally motivated adaptive conflicts constitute the primary motivations in psychic conflict and that their resolution constitutes a certain level of healing. In contrast, Jung does not admit the strong split between adaptive and psychodynamic or outer and inner dimensions of an adaptive situation. Rather there is a multiplicity of motivations for Jung, consciously pertaining to the adaptive conflict but also in some measure, below the surface, pertaining the basic teleological impulse toward wholeness and thus toward developing hitherto unconscious functions, functional ranges, or rendering complexes conscious. On Jung's account, therefore, what at the level of immediate consciousness Langs would call an "adaptive context" or "trigger" (for psychic conflict), Jung would say is *also* an outer occasion of an inner motivation, rooted in the psyche's teleological drive, to develop relatively unconscious dimensions of the psyche. This set of issues will be developed in more detail later in this chapter.

Since adaptive issues, for both Langs and Jung, play such a central role in clinical practices such as understanding unconscious communication, recognizing the sources of psychic conflict, and aiding in the restoration of a balance of consciousness in a patient, we can draw the probable conclusion that both Langs and Jung would most likely agree that adaptation requires a special and consistent focus in all clinical interaction. This conclusion is beyond question in the case of Langs, who stakes all clinical understanding on adaptation. But we would further suggest that Jung, who does not write clinically focused texts in the manner of Langs and so will not necessarily have the same occasions to emphasize this point, would in principle agree with the thesis himself. Furthermore, referring back to the introduction and the problem of adaptation as a field of motivation, we could add that other Jungian approaches in some measure require the recognition of adaptive problems, even when their method is focused on archetypes and other generalized phenomena typical to Jungian practice. For example, an archetypal approach can be deeply illuminating of concrete material, such as Jung's brilliant analyses in the last of the *Tavistock Lectures* (Jung, 1968). However, such an approach to clinical phenomena—as Jung himself illustrates in the *Lectures*—is not really a highlighting the material *in its concreteness* but rather understanding of that material in terms of broader narratives and analogies rooted in the commonality of human nature and cultural generalities (i.e., archetypally). The point being emphasized here, therefore, is not to reduce the value of an archetypal approach but only to recognize that an archetypal approach is not a substitute for the particularities and concreteness of the clinical material and its quite specific and particular adaptive focus in a given case and situation. Indeed, as we have tried to show, those same concrete factors also condition which of the potentialities contained in archetypal material refers to this patient, in the here and now.

Langs' own development of the adaptive paradigm was partially in response to his feeling that purely intrapsychic approaches to material among psychoanalysts often ended up looking like the free associations of the analyst, rather than material derived from and relevant to the patient. A Jungian might fall into a very similar trap if one conflates an archetypal approach to material as a substitute for the concrete, adaptive approach, because the tendency would be simply to focus on the *possible* illuminations of the material in terms of archetypes, rather than how it *actually* illuminates the material in a specific, concrete, and adaptive situation.

How Langs and Jung Might Supplement Each Other

While Langs and Jung do share some important orientations and sensibilities with each other, there are at least as many points of difference as there are points of similarity. Some of these differences pertain to distinct—sometimes incompatible—conceptions of the psyche, a point to which we will return in the next section. At other times, their individual conceptions of adaptation can each be interpreted as supplementing the other, as if focusing on different elements of adaptation and how adaptive issues impact the clinical setting. This point was illustrated in some measure in chapter 4, where some of the same clinical material used for a Langsian approach was also used for understanding Jung's approach. At this point, we need to understand why both approaches can be used simultaneously.

Langs' consistent picture of adaptation throughout his forty years of developing the idea focuses on what we might call "moments" in the clinical process or, more precisely, "moments" in a clinical session. The term "moments" is here used to refer to brief episodes in any given session which seem to form discrete and meaningful units. By using the term "moments," we are basically using a heuristic fiction by which to imagine what is essentially a process, the therapeutic process, as if it were divided into discrete pieces—snapshots, if you will—each a meaningful unit. In Langs' theory and virtually always in his clinical illustrations, adaptive contexts are posed in terms of such moments (e.g., brief vignettes or small pieces of dialogue from a session) and are characteristically defined, as we would expect, in terms of some event external to the patient's psyche to which a patient is adapting. This approach to clinical material and illustrations is in some measure demanded by Langs' assumption that adaptation refers to aspects of clinical material that are so concrete that essentially each new moment or "snapshot" in the process amounts to a new adaptive context, both in what the patient is describing (adaptation to the world) and in what is occurring in the session (adaptation in the therapeutic relationship). Once that adaptive context is recognized as such, Langs tends to think that the material in the session can be related to that context and delineated, in principle, as to its unconscious meaning. In Langs' understanding of the clinical situation, the insights gained from these discrete moments, whereby specific events are read as adaptive contexts and psychic conflict is linked to those contexts, is basically what the work of psychoanalytic therapy consists in, something which the patient finds, as Langs frequently puts it, "deeply healing."

There appears no good reason to deny this basic thrust in Langs' work, and the case of Bruce in chapter 3 was offered to illustrate a more or less successful use of Langs' methods. Yet we should also note that, true to Langs' style, the illustration offered in chapter 3 focuses on a few particular moments in the treatment which express specific derivatively communicated themes (nosy supervisors, ways of getting around boss' expectations, and so forth), which in turn indicate both psychic conflict and an adaptive context (in this case unconscious conflict of having the tape recorder in the room). This approach to the material did indeed produce insight into unconscious communications and offer, in the end, relief to the patient, especially once Bruce recognized that the tape recorder both could and should be removed from the room (the adaptive context), so that he could speak freely and without fear, concerning his material.

Nonetheless, it appears that Langs confuses the part for the whole, emphasizing one element of adaptively charged meaning in the clinical session and one element of psychoanalytic method, to the point of missing other at least equally important aspects which Jung highlights, such as the fundamental changes in a person's overall orientation toward life through attitudinal shifts and functional change and expansion. Among Langs' strength as a writer and a researcher is his ability to analyze clinical experiences into smaller, discrete moments, and to recognize each of these as meaningful units. These units and their derivatively communicated links appear to be the core of Langs' interests and to comprise, for Langs, the essence of therapeutic change, in that insight into adaptive issues in these moments brings longer term understanding and healing.

Unfortunately, Langs' ability to *analyze* sessions into smaller units does not seem to have been complemented by an equal ability to *synthesize* those discrete parts into a picture of the overall trajectory which delineates how discrete adaptive moments might serve some larger psychological perspective, process, or whole. Indeed, Langs might even doubt that there is some larger process to be served, perhaps being satisfied that symptom relief and insight into how one must adapt to therapy or to specific life events as sufficient goals of psychoanalytic psychotherapy. If this suspicion is on target, it would highlight a substantial difference between Langs' view and that of Jung.

In contrast to Langs' style of thinking, Jung's development of adaptation in *On Psychic Energy* does not include much by way of clinical moments of the sort Langs uses more or less exclusively, in part because no such moment *could* illustrate the point Jung is making. Adaptation in Jung's sense refers to how inner changes in the broad psychic orientations and functions occur as well as potentially shorter-term but nonetheless long-range changes regarding one's relationships to one's own complexes, something which can only be illustrated by a description of a longer process, since such change would only very rarely if ever occur in a single clinical moment. From this point of view, one might object that Langs' tendency always to illustrate by means of clinical moment, though certainly having its virtues, may also hide the fact that he is in practice reducing adaptation to one—and not necessarily or always the most important—component. Rather, some elements of the analytic process are perhaps not simply the sum of discrete adaptive problems and their psychological solutions. If we follow Jung on this point, we must admit that there are what we might term "structural" features of the individual psyche, including various energetically and emotionally charged and partially unconscious psychic nodes—what Jung calls "complexes"— and also long-term functional and attitudinal orientations, which can also be reoriented. Further, there is a teleological direction intrinsic to the human psyche which, though expressing itself uniquely in the personality and history of the patient, nonetheless codetermines the specific psychic conflicts that one has at any given moment. As we saw in the last chapter, according to Jung, the regression of libido or psychic energy occurs because the active, dominant function cannot resolve the outer problem and hence demands some development of the more latent and unconscious function which can resolve the problem. For Jung, both the adaptive issues and the unconscious elements we seek to understand, articulate, and interpret are themselves bound up with what we have termed "structural" features of the psyche and its inner dynamism which impels it to move toward wholeness.

This discussion illuminates the fact that there seems no inherent reason for us to choose Langs' or Jung's approach at the expense of the other and this for at least two reasons: (1) because at least some of the same case material and same methods (e.g., interpreting derivative communication) seem to indicate two distinct forms or levels of adaptation, at we saw in the case of Bruce, both of which may at least potentially serve psychological healing and wholeness and neither of which seem inherently to exclude the other: Langs' approach referring to the *concrete, historical events* of a patient's life and (mal)adaptive responses to them, Jung referring to the ongoing *development and expansion of psychic energy and psychic structure* of the patient through responding to adaptive contexts; (2) since the analytic materials and methods used seem to coalesce around *both* forms of adaptation, it is safe to assume that they are connected and in some sense "meant" to be understood together. How they might be understood together is, at this point, not terribly mysterious.

Langs' approach focuses on the immediate adaptive issues and how some level of psychological change is necessary in order for one to respond adequately to immediate adaptive contexts. However, Langs does not offer much by way of general contextual directions *in psychic life itself* for what counts as adaptive gains (or losses) for the patient. There are many reasons Langs does not do this, some of which are questions of principle for him. For one, Langs' focus is invariably on the patient's unconscious communications—and these alone—for guiding the analytic and interpretive work of the analyst or therapist. One does not find in Langs much by way of structural articulations of the psyche and he all but rejects the use of complex theory. As his work develops, in fact, Langs considered Freud's structural model of the psyche to be a central ground for all that was wrong in the psychoanalytic tradition (Langs, 1992). When, in his later work, he evidently feels some need to articulate something of a theory of psychic structure to ground his clinical theory (Langs, 2004a), the latter is used exclusively as an explanatory model for why trauma and death anxiety are the fundamental causes of psychic conflict: so far as this reader can tell the psychic structure Langs develops does not enter into his actual clinical considerations, other than the theoretical separation of the "unconscious," which contains repressed or denied contents, and the "deep unconscious," which is the unconscious wisdom system informing the analyst or therapist of the psychological needs of the patient (Langs, 2004). Consequently, it appears that Langs intended psychoanalytic clinical method to consist more or less exclusively in reading the individual unconscious communications of the patient in the immediate adaptive context, without reference to anything structural or any direction of structural change of the individual psyche. This point does not seem fundamentally to change throughout his life and is one consistent principle from the inception of Langs' adaptive thinking.

Furthermore, because of the exclusive primacy of unconscious communication in Langs' clinical approach, he has a certain aversion to what he would term "conscious-level" inferences about the meaning of material, especially the kind of inference that is heavily theory laden. Always at heart an empiricist, Langs was convinced that psychoanalytic practice in recent decades had essentially eschewed the central task of psychoanalysis, namely, aiding the patient interpretatively through understanding unconscious communications. For this reason, Langs consistently avoided much by way of talk about psychic structure, outside of forming a set of theoretical assumptions, generally opting for very concrete analyses of particular adaptive problems and drawing general clinical principles from this material.

However, this focus in Langs leaves open the question of the psychological value of adaptation: does highlighting adaptive issues in therapy simply allow one to focus on unconscious communication and symptom relief or is there something more essential to psychic life that adaptive issues are in the service of? Without some clear sense of a teleology in the psyche (or something of equivalent significance and meaning-conferring ability), the former answer is largely unavoidable. In contrast, based on the analysis of Jung, it appears adaptation is potentially a more formidable principle of analytic work than even Langs admitted.

Adaptation, as it is articulated in Jung, supplies some of the structural features which can confer meaning on discrete adaptive moments and situations, by contextualizing them as part of a long-term and purely psychological process. Because Jung does not separate the "externally" adaptive and the "internally" psychic (or psychodynamic) dimensions of the adaptive situation, he can *both* acknowledge the particular adaptive contexts and the concrete needs for adaptation to an environment *and* potentially recognize these discrete adaptive moments as part of a larger movement toward the expansion of attitudinal and functional material as well as an increase of available psychic energy, due to the rendering of unconscious aspects of the psyche more conscious.

Furthermore, Jung's analysis can partially supply two implicit premises for Langs' theory that Langs did not seem to recognize he needed to articulate: (1) that any adaptive change would seem to require some increase in psychic energy, and (2) that any recognition of the need to change would presume an experience of a value hierarchy. Concerning the first point, presumably a patient who needs to change the manner in which they are adapting must also elicit a certain quantum of energy, both to liberate oneself from old adaptive habits and in order to develop a new way of adapting. It would appear to be an insufficient analysis of the adaptive issue, therefore, simply to note the outer adaptive trigger and recognize the need to change: change typically requires acting outside one's established comfort zone and being willing to do what does not come easy. Jung's theory suggests both that the energy dammed up by the adaptive task and adaptive impasse can be transformed and also that, typically, some new quantum of energy from the unconscious is elicited by the adaptive process. Consequently, it is intrinsic to the adaptive process that there is both an increase as well as a transformation of energy, at least if adaptation is successful (Jung, 1955). Now Langs might consider that a purely theoretical point and of no real importance clinically. In contrast, as we discussed in chapter 4, Jung would use this point clinically, by looking to where there appears to be quantitative energy shifts and where new potentials are emerging in the patient's material, both in dream and phantasy images as well as in observation in sessions.

Concerning the second point, though Jung does not have a robust value theory, he does think that the feeling function as well as broader emotioxperiences have reference to value. As was pointed out last chapter, the "feeling function" for Jung consists among other things in the ability to experience values and "affect," though not the feeling function per se, also implies a certain emotional relationship to value because it is conceived in terms of being appropriate or inappropriate, suggesting that affect is measured in terms of value: does it "fit" to the occasion or is it "harmonious" or "consonant" with what is demanded or not; or, in other words, *is it adaptive?* Thus, adaptation and the emotional energy associated with it characteristically includes an implicit experience of value and of a rank order of those values, something our analyses of both Freud and Hartmann in chapter 2 also suggested. Jung does not develop the points concerning value, to be sure, since his interest is in the psychological factors and not in the external value factors, yet the underlying assumption for his understanding of both the feeling function and affect is a recognition of value—value in an objective, external world sense.

Here Max Scheler might aid in our understanding of Jung's point, Scheler being the premier value philosopher of his time, just when Jung is developing his theory of the psychological types. Following Scheler on value experience (Scheler, 1973; Scheler, 1973a; White, forthcoming), we can say that, typically, values are not experienced as individual, discrete entities; in contrast, when we examine carefully our experience of values, they are usually experienced in terms of an implicit hierarchy or rank order. The ranking of values, in fact, is often so automatic or taken for granted that one often doesn't recognize that such ranking is typically intrinsic to the experience of value, whether the value is of great importance in one's life or not. It might take the form of experiencing an excellent concert but implicitly noting the band did a better job the previous time, or realizing that one enjoys black raspberry ice cream more than cherry but not as much strawberry, or at a deeper level that one loves one's father, but that he could have done a better job in some specific ways. In each of these cases, there is both the recognition of a value and an implicit recognition of the *value context*, such that values are experienced, as a rule, within a rank order of higher and lower and this rank order is in fact an aspect of the original value experience.

This point matters not only theoretically but also clinically when it comes to treating adaptive issues, because value issues almost invariably set the context of the adaptive trigger. As we have seen, Jung's analysis suggesting that adaptive issues always provoke pent-up affect (or the lack of affect) already indicates a value context for adaptation, because of the value assumption of whether the affect "fits" or is "appropriate" to the situation. Furthermore, standard adaptive triggers as a rule suggest that value and value experiences are intrinsic to them, such as problems associated with leaving once-beneficial environments for new ones as in a marriage or career situation (the former being experienced as a lower, the latter a higher value), dropping old positive or negative idealizations about significant others (idealizations clearly imply value), or allowing oneself to feel the pain of trauma in order to work through it in order to feel more alive after (i.e., it is worth struggling psychologically with something value-negative, like traumatic experiences, in order to come to the higher positive value of feeling more alive). In each of these quite typical therapeutic situations there is at least an implicit experience of value and value ranks and, as a rule, no movement away from avoidance and toward a better adaptation will occur until the patient allows the experience and the feeling of attraction toward the higher value to aid and encourage the development of a new adaptive style—especially when the new adaptation requires what Hartmann calls "detours" (i.e., the psychologically challenging and emotionally risky business of a hit and miss process [Hartmann, 1958]).

Hence, while there is a good deal of merit in Langs' assessment of adaptive issues and in his analysis of adaptive problems in terms of clinical moments, he has no clear way of interpreting those discrete moments in terms of a larger and distinctively psychological context, which articulates in a meaningful way how distinct adaptive events and clinical moments result is an overall psychological development and expansion of psychic life, let alone an expansion of value experience—just what Jung's theory in some measure supplies. Jung's understanding of adaptation can countenance virtually every point that Langs develops, including the significance of derivatives for unconscious communication (as we saw last chapter), while also understanding the basic movement toward functional and energic expansion. Hence, Jung's approach, rather than excluding Langs' often brilliant technical moves, can include much of his approach while also adding something missing to Langs' view, namely, a longer-term and thoroughly psychological ground for adaptation, a ground which is more than merely the psyche's response to external triggers, and the beginnings of a theory of how both psychic energy and value experience expand.

From a technical standpoint, therefore, Langs is very much on target in his conviction that adaptive issues are central both to psychic conflict and to understanding unconscious communication. Furthermore, as we saw last chapter, we can in principle use Langs' listening-intervening-validating method well beyond the context of clinical moments also for the recognition of more directional adaptive change. Hence, technically speaking, some formulation of adaptive problems should be kept in mind by the analyst or therapist, especially when the clinical material indicates psychic conflict in need of resolution and especially, as in Jung, when some imbalance or inappropriate affect (too much or too little) appears to emerge in adaptively charged situations. However, we add to Langs' understanding that there is also an overall and structural dimension to adaptation, which requires a sense of where the teleology of the patient's psyche and of the therapeutic process as a whole is leading. This teleology is not the mere generalization that the psyche seeks wholeness but is rather a concretely indicated movement of the individual psyche, discovered *within* adaptive contexts. Recognizing, therefore, where the patient appears either to be stuck due to unconscious complexes or to indicate regression of energy due to functional or attitudinal limitations, is just as essential to understanding clinical and adaptive material as the particular external adaptive trigger. The adaptive issue is, on this account, *never* exclusively about adapting within the given outer environment and adaptive problems posed by the patient in a concrete moment; there is rather *always also* an issue of the expansion of psychic resources which can in some measure be defined through alterations in unconscious complexes and underdeveloped psychic functions and attitudes. These points, derived from Jung, can help the analyst recognize not only the adaptive problems and resolutions in Langs' sense but also where the patient's psyche needs development and expansion, including from the standpoint of value experience. Indeed, from a clinical standpoint, it is in principle always an option which aspect of adaptation to focus on, that which Langs' develops or that which Jung develops, something which one generally discerns through evaluating the existing indications in the session.

At this point, it should be noted that Langs would quite likely *not* find either this attempt at expanding adaptive issues into a structural dimension of the psyche or the attempt in chapter 4 of interpreting case material in these ways satisfactory, for at least the two reasons already given: (1) he would consider the chapter 4 interpretation of material to be primarily *inferential* rather than given through the process of listening-intervening-validating that he underlines throughout his work, and (2) he would further consider such inferences—those associated with structural features of the psyche—primarily or exclusively *conscious level* considerations, rather than properly unconscious communications. Hence, our proposed linking of Langs and Jung would very likely appear to Langs as appeasing what he views as the unfortunate tendencies in contemporary psychoanalysis toward conscious-level approaches.

At least the following might be given in immediate response to this imagined objection from Langs: there is no reason to think that the appropriate analytic method for elucidating moments and their unconscious meanings would also be appropriate for the task of understanding these psychic reorientations; different kinds of phenomena generally require different sorts of methods and approaches. Thus, the imagined objection from Langs assumes a singular method for analytic practice or a singular method for analysis of all aspects of the psyche, a premise that Jung (and certainly this author) would not accept. Given this latter point, one could respond to Langs directly simply by saying that it is true that Jung's approach to complexes as well as to functional and attitudinal change is different from any focus that emphasizes clinical moments exclusively. Yet that is just what we would expect since these are two different strata or levels of psychic life. Langs confuses the part for the whole.

Incompatibilities between Langs and Jung

Nonetheless, such a response would not penetrate to the deeper differences between Langs and Jung, especially if our goal is to illuminate the potential value each has clinically when it comes to understanding and interpreting adaptation. We can begin to see these deeper differences if we consider the extent to which their relevant theories of the psyche impact their conceptions of clinical material.

Characteristic of Langs' clinical approach is the lack of sense for what Jung called the "reality of the psyche" (a point highlighted in both chapters 1 and 3), whereby Langs focuses almost exclusively on the products of the psyche, such as fantasies, images, symbols, memories, etc. Because of his contention of the reality of the psyche, Jung quite logically reads clinical material not only as *products* of the psyche but also as *expressions* of individual psychic structure, such as complexes, functions, and general attitudes. Langs displays little or no sense for what Jung means by "psychic reality" and in fact is amazingly free of meaningful references to complexes for someone who prides himself on working within the "classical psychoanalytic tradition." In our personal correspondence, Langs wrote explicitly that he never saw much value to complex theory.

This basic difference between Langs and Jung seems to entail the primary difference in their reading of adaptation. Langs' lack of feeling for psychic reality in Jung's sense seems the primary reason why his work on adaptation must focus more or less exclusively on specific moments in the therapeutic process and on particular, external events: precisely the longer-lasting elements of psychic reality, such as complexes, functions, and attitudes have no real place in Langs' theory, which cannot countenance the psyche as a reality of its own; Langs appears not to feel this lack. His development of adaptation must therefore focus where it does, with discrete moments and external events. In contrast, Jung's recognition of psychic reality permits a vision of the psyche and of adaptation that recognizes longer lasting stances and attitudes of the person and how they modify in and through the discrete events that Langs focuses on.

Furthermore, this difference entails further clinical differences between Langs and Jung, some of which by necessity impact how they would treat adaptation in clinical contexts. For one, the lack of psychic reality or some surrogate for it in Langs' theory means that, among other things, there is nothing like teleology in his theory: if there's no psyche outside its products, there is no teleology of the psyche. Jung, in contrast, believes that he can read something of that teleology in all the products of the psyche and thus, for example, insists on the possibility of "prospective" interpretations of symbols, something Langs' theory as such cannot admit (though a Jungian integrating Langs' theory could include this in principle). This cannot but impact the understanding of adaptation, especially if the previous suggestion that adaptation operationalizes teleology is correct. For Langs, adaptation must simply be a consequence of our being organisms, since there appears to be no psychic reality outside of our being living matter; for Jung, adaptation is certainly an aspect of our being organisms, but it is *also* expressive of a kind of psychological destiny to wholeness. For Langs, psychological insight into adaptive problems is basically "healing" because it relieves symptoms. For Jung, psychological insight into adaptive problems can certainly lead to healing one's symptoms but, more importantly, acts as a clue to how one's destiny toward wholeness is to be achieved. We might add here that Langs seems to understand adaptation more in terms of a state—one is relieved of the psychological consequences of maladaptation—rather than as a process, as Jung clearly sees it. From a technical standpoint, each of these can illuminate the other, but neither should be understood as the whole.

We just used the somewhat dramatic language of "destiny" to discuss adaptive issues quite purposely, because there is an "existential" side to adaptation that these points imply. If adaptive issues are as much at the heart of analytic process as we are saying and, even more importantly, if they are as much at the heart of the life process and the process of individuation as this all suggests, then issues of adaptation are expressive of human destiny (i.e., the destiny of each individual human being to become as whole as possible). Though this might appear to be an overly dramatic statement, working with any patient who can't seem to get out of a basic "stuckness," a patient for whom a new form of adaptation appears impossible or who feels condemned to a repetition compulsion, will convince one otherwise. In the latter case, what ideally would be a feeling of destiny toward wholeness is missing and any talk about individuation feels like a promised land to which the patient can never arrive; indeed, a promised land which, unlike Moses, the patient can never even see. As Jung put it in various contexts, when the unconscious is not made conscious, life appears as a kind fate, as if it is necessitated and could never have been different. Destiny, in contrast, is the feeling and experience of life's potential, whereas fate is the feeling and experience that there is no potential, that life merely "happens" to one, rather than a cooperative cocreation between one's capacity to choose and one's general teleological impulses. Adaptive problems, perhaps more than any other experience, bring with them the existential question of whether life is fate or destiny.

Returning to the imagined objections of Langs to Jung raised in the last section, such that Jung's treatment of adaptation is too inferential and too conscious level, the previous points should give us a feeling of the response Jung might make. First of all, any assumption that complexes, functional directions, or attitudinal differences are mere "theory" would certainly be rejected by Jung. As Jung makes quite clear through his work with the Word Association Test as well as his work on the psychological types, he believes all these psychic dimensions are empirically established and to some degree observable in one's patients, especially over time. Jung would not admit the substantial gap between empirical data and theory that Langs assumes, the latter arising from Langs' tendency we alluded to in chapter 3 to use the hard sciences as his model.

Jung would probably further respond by saying that illuminating unconscious material is not per se the end-all and be-all of analytic therapy; rather, the goal of analytic work is aiding the individuation pro-cess of the patient. Hence, Jung would not assume that if something is "conscious level," it is not of analytic significance. Similarly, Jung would probably also deny that references to structural features of the psyche amount to "mere inferences" about unconscious communications. After all, if one is going to understand the significant unconscious material to be structural, as Jung does, presumably one needs to understand something about the patient's conscious psychic structure to understand what in the patient's psychic structure requires development. Such a move would not seem to this author to be significantly different from, say, looking at conscious-level problems as indicators of adaptive issues and then reading the unconscious material accordingly—Langs' stated method of approach. In both cases, some hypotheses of what is going are made based on the observation of conscious-level experiences and the reading of unconscious material is achieved in part in the light of those hypotheses, not outside of them.

Finally, as pointed out last chapter, one can also use Langs' listening-intervening-validating model to confirm which structural dimensions of the psyche are in need of development. That one's general sense of typology, for example, might be based on observation in no way implies that one ought not also look for unconscious communications to verify one's observations. Quite the contrary, the case of Bruce demonstrated ways in which one could use Langs' method to confirm observed structural deficits in the patient.

For this reason, there appears no cogent reason to assume that Langs' distinctive way of listening-intervening-validating could not apply to Jung's understanding of adaptation, just because the latter is based in part on structure rather than on concrete history. Far from being "mere inferences," the structural factors that Jung offers can act as guideposts to aid the analyst in recognizing where adaptation and maladaptation are or are likely to be taking place and how adaptive and maladaptive contents (Langs) and pro-cesses (Jung) indicated in the unconscious material might be interpreted and understood. Typical to Jung's approach, some understanding of the underly-ing commonalities in human nature (expressed earlier all in myth and arche-typal material) are just as important for understanding clinical material as the specific symbols and contents of an individual psyche, precisely because not all psychic conflict is exclusively born of the concrete historical factors in the person: some psychic conflict arises from underdeveloped psychic functioning and unconscious complexes, which are common denominators in human nature and are not as a rule exclusively functions of particular adaptive or maladaptive events. Just as Jung's sense for human nature in gen-eral allows for an archetypal reading of material, so it also allows for struc-tural and complex-based interpretations of material (Jung, 1954).

Hence, with regard to understanding the structure of the individual psyche and its role in understanding clinical material, it would appear that one cannot be both a Langsian and a Jungian. For Langs, structural fea-tures are considered too exclusively theoretical to enter validly into clinical material and thus, for example, the reading of Bruce's money issue as something related to the feeling function due to the value symbol would no doubt seem to Langs far too theoretical and inferential to be valid. In contrast, from a more properly Jungian point of view, one of the things one would expect of the psyche is that its unconscious psychic communications are always also speaking about the psyche itself (i.e., about its own long-term development, not only about the contingent historical events that pose adaptive problems). Once this point is granted, it appears further that the listening-intervening-validating technique of Langs is in principle applicable to unconscious material and communication also when we are looking at structurally based adaptation, as in fact I did with the case of Bruce. Whereas a purely Langsian approach must exclude most of these Jungian points, the Jungian can include the Langsian points as valid technical contributions and expand them into areas where Langs would likely not have gone, while nonetheless granting that Jung's approach to adaptation is only a part of a clinical whole, to which Langs' understanding contributes a good deal.

Understanding Symbols

Their differing conceptions and assumptions about human nature imply more clinical differences between Langs and Jung than I have hitherto suggested. Among the most important and clinically relevant differences regard the nature and function of symbols.

In chapter 3 we developed Langs' differentiation among three communicative fields. We saw there that the simplest and most direct way of differentiating the fields is in terms of the relationship of the ego to affective and emotional life: the Type C or persona-restoring field implying a lack of conscious linking to affect, Type B or complex-discharging field implying being too immersed in affect and discharging it, and Type A or secured-symbolizing field implying a conscious and contained relationship to affect. For Langs the Type A or secured-symbolizing field is the ideal case for the expression of unconscious material. In his later work, Langs holds to essentially the same view, though focusing on how narrative or story telling is the primary (or perhaps exclusive) communicative vehicle for the Type A field.

This differentiation helps bring into focus one reason why the three distinct communicative fields can best be defined in terms of ego and affect. Following Jung on this point, we can say that a key indicator of adaptive problems is inappropriate affect, where "inappropriate" can mean either too much or too little affect in relation to the adaptive issue at hand. Consequently, only when the affect, along with its inadequate measure, can also be contained psychologically and brought into relatively conscious relationship to the ego, can we expect to do full-blown analytic work. Lack of connection to affect (Type C) or lack of ability to contain it (Type B) more or less guarantees that adequate symbolization will not occur.

It is perhaps this aspect of the interactive field, more than any other, which convinced Langs of the importance of the "frame" of psychotherapy. Langs spent a good deal of ink in the 1970s and 1980s attempting to define the conditions under which the Type A or secured-symbolizing field could obtain, and this particular aspect of Langs' work never fundamentally changed, once he recognized it. Even in his final book on technique (Langs, 2004), Langs offers more than a dozen characteristics of the ideal, secured frame which guarantees, he thinks, a secured-symbolizing field, to the extent one conforms to it. As with most of the discussions of Langs in this chapter, we would accept Langs' basic points as far as they go. However, we would also posit that Langs has again conflated the part he has seen clearly with the whole, especially with regard to two things: (1) Langs' conception of symbol appears to be limited to *linguistic* symbol, and (2) Langs' "frame" cannot itself be symbolized.

Concerning the first point, Langs appears very much to assume the idea that analytic work is "talk therapy," focusing almost exclusively on linguistic communication as the vehicle for therapeutic work. Indeed, for a brief period, Langs' gave up the name "adaptive" approach for his style of therapy in favor of the "communicative approach" or "communicative psychotherapy," emphasizing thereby the importance of language and of reading the unconscious through derivative communications. The communicative fields that Langs develops are all about linguistic communication and the nature of those communications in each of the fields, thus showing how much a philosophy of language is at the basis of Langs' theory. And yet it seems significant that, however important derivative communication is for understanding unconscious communications—and it *is* important—it by no means exhausts the ways in which the unconscious is manifest in the warp and woof of a session. Langs appears to isolate a very significant point, namely how and why derivative communication works to illuminate unconscious processes, but also seems to unduly restrict symbolization to such communications.

There's good reason, as pointed out in chapter 3, to think that not everything in an image can be so directly translated into language: language works best with images when it circumambulates the image through amplification, comparisons, contrasts, and the like. The reason for this is that language and linguistic practice generally—unless it is drawn from a partially unconscious state, such as reverie—trends toward clarity and univocity, whereas images are by nature multivalent, many-layered, multi-colored. It is rarely the case that a term or sentence adequately captures a symbol or image by itself, precisely because these characteristics of language contrast to the nature of symbols and images. Hence it is not obvious that typical language and linguistic communication themselves are either sufficient or the best paradigms for how we understand unconscious material and productions of images and symbols. This point seems also to be true from an evolutionary standpoint: the unconscious pre-existed consciousness;

hence the "language" of the unconscious—images and symbols (along with affect)—probably predated the verbal language of consciousness and, presumably, has at least some differences of purpose and function.

Furthermore, many times what count as "symbols" are simply not linguistic, even if they can be pointed to or indicated by language. Bruce and I ritually turning off the tape recorder is certainly symbolic, for both of us, and meaningful as a gesture.[5] Its multivalence also comes through when we consider the two different readings we gave to it in chapters 3 and 4: the first as a ritual surrender of what was inhibiting communication between us, the second as a symbol of giving up an "external" recorder and turning to Bruce's "internal" recorder (i.e., his memories of the painful feelings which burdened him so deeply and which he avoided as much as he could). While we certainly can point to that symbolic action via language, as was done just now by describing the situation, the description is not the symbol; the gesture is the embodied symbol. If one reduces the latter to the former, one basically denudes the event of its psychological force and multivalent meaning, treating it as little more than an occasion for univocal language. Indeed, this specific aspect of Langs' work is somewhat ironic: after all, Langs emphasized the "reality" of the external adaptive context, in contrast to the mere "fantasy" of the products of the psyche, such as psychic images. Yet here there appears a reduction of what one might consider a "real symbol," such as the gesture of turning off the tape recorder, to a model of symbol in language, something that, as a product of the psyche, one would think as having far less "reality" in Langs' sense.

If one reads carefully through Langs' literally hundreds of clinical vignettes, one will almost invariably find that imagistic and symbolic entities as a rule get translated out of their multivalence and into literalistic statements, by which Langs seeks to aid the patient to understand their psychic conflict with insight. Such reductions can be valuable and are always permitted in analytic practice, providing we not lose the fact that such an approach is really a reduction and that the symbol or image by nature contains more implications than we are saying (Kugler and Hillman, 1985).

But one sees very little of the latter in Langs, who seems content to translate images and symbols into straightforward language, a habit of mind which suggests significant problems for understanding the symbol. For it seems to say that the symbol always has the character of a means to an end. Langs never seems to treat the productions of symbols by the psyche as ends in themselves, rather seeing them purely as means for psychological understanding that need to be unraveled and decoded. For example, for Langs, we try to gain a secured-symbolizing field not first and foremost to encourage the patient to symbolize per se, but so we can interpret those symbols in basically non-symbolic, "decoded" ways.

---

5. Goodheart (1980) also offers an example of a gesture (in his case, a patient wanting to stand up and walk around the room) and its symbolic meaning.

This aspect of Langs' approach, combined with his focus more or less exclusively on clinical moments, in essence de-symbolizes the symbol. The multivalence of symbols is not an accident of psychic life but something the psyche does in order to connect aspects of psychic life and experience that cannot be linked meaningfully through cause and effect and other sets of cognitive and rational relationships. Jung's analysis in the "The Transcendent Function" is very much to the point: the symbol links apparent opposites into a single unity through its multivalence, allowing for seemingly incompatible factors to be linked into meaningful unities. Thus, the symbol of the tape recorder in Bruce's case, for example, linked together Bruce's need for privacy and respect for his material, on the one hand, with his somewhat repressed feeling function, on the other. Such unconsciously produced symbols tend, if anything, to be overdetermined by a number of potential meanings, which decoding into singular and literal language vehicles can in principle illuminate but equally obscure. While Langs would probably not deny the multivalence of symbols, his method appears to literalize symbols into singular, linguistically expressed meanings.

This point in fact may help elucidate the second criticism mentioned earlier, concerning the analytic frame. For Langs, the frame is conceived of as a condition of symbolizing, for reasons outlined in chapter 3. However, it does not seem to have occurred to Langs that the frame itself is ultimately a symbol and, in fact, should become a living part of the secured-symbolizing field between analyst and patient. For one, the language of "frame" is by no means the only language one might use; "holding," for example, has been a common symbol used for the frame in the psychoanalytic tradition and "container" in the Jungian (Cwik, 2010), each having very different imagistic implications from "frame." Yet all three appear to be valid characterizations of the therapeutic context. Hence, it appears that Langs literalized his favored symbol into something of a straitjacket, losing other potentially valuable metaphors.[6] Further, as Jung suggests, a symbol is never *merely* a means to some other end, even if it can be a means as well. As we saw in chapter 4, the symbol has the power to unite opposites; the symbol is therefore what heals because it can encompass and unite the dualities of being and experience: conscious and unconscious, I and thou, opposing psychological functions, introversion and extraversion, and the like, into a kind of equilibrium. Symbols are neither surrogates for what can be said better in literal terms, nor are they simply means in order to gain something else. One might say the entire point of analysis for Jung is to learn to live a *symbolic life*, in order that symbolic multivalence can confer

---

6. Kugler and Hillman (1985) highlight an interesting irony in this use of the frame metaphor in the case of Goodheart (though it applies equally well to Langs). On the one hand, the metaphor can become unconscious enough to control uncritically the entire discourse around analytic structure (e.g., talk about "frame violations," "maintaining the frame," etc.) and yet, on the other hand, be treated in a purely literal way, as if those latter metaphors are literal statements.

a unitary meaning on diverse yet psychologically connected experiences.[7] Though Hartmann does not speak in his essay on adaptation of the role of symbolization in psychological life, it is clear that Jung's interests in symbol here are close to Hartmann's concerns about finding various psychological equilibriums, discussed in chapter 2.

Contrast that relatively rigid Langsian view of the frame to the view at least implicit in Jung's *Psychology of the Transference* where, in the *Rosarium* plates, the King and Queen are in the bath together (i.e. where the frame *itself*, imaged in the fountain in which they bathe, becomes just as much a part of the symbolic field as the pair themselves [Cwik, 2006; Cwik, 2010; Cwik, 2011; Cwik, 2017]). This image, as interpreted by Jung and by Cwik, represents the way the frame is taken into the communicative field and becomes lived in the therapeutic relationship. The symbolic life is expressed in the ability of a person to live alternatives in a kind of differentiated unity, rather than repressing or suppressing one side of the opposition. In the case of the frame, for example, Langs may be correct that the frame should be secure and literal—and *external*—at the beginning of treatment, suggesting a kind of opposite of security (limit), on the one hand, and freedom to symbolize (lack of limit), on the other. But in practice, isn't the goal of the secure frame that it become internalized and intrinsic to the therapeutic relationship, so that the patient (and analyst) no longer needs an external frame to keep the symbolizing field intact because the frame has been internalized as a conscious, self-limiting principle, for which each party is responsible? It would seem the frame works best when it becomes symbolically enacted in the therapeutic relationship and becomes a lived, psychological phenomenon by which the patient takes full responsibility for their psychological process, rather than simply being responsive (or worse reactive) to the analyst's or therapist's external demands.[8]

If this point is correct, we can see one of the limits of Langs' insistence on adaptive factors being always external stimuli. Because he insists on the sharp distinction between outer adaptive contexts and inner psychic reactions to them, Langs must in principle always keep important adaptive triggers in the outer world. If, instead, we do not accept the sharp differentiation between inner and outer that Langs presumes, but also recognize that some outer adaptive factors need to become inner, psychological factors, we can also see that the sharp differentiation of inner and outer in Langs may not always be beneficial to healthy adaptation.

While these points are in one sense quite general, they apply quite directly to the problem of adaptation. Langs' development of adaptation suggests an approach to the psyche which respects external adaptive contexts insofar as

---

7. The significance of symbols and their multivalence go well beyond individual psychology into understanding the ties that bind social, political, and religious communities. For example, see White (2011) regarding the importance of symbol for a religious and theological problem.

8. Gill (1984) also notes that patients may not want or need to be "held" in the same way, something which Langs' relatively rigid conception of the frame cannot countenance.

the latter pose psychic conflict but by treating symbols as mere means to resolving the conflict, the symbols themselves potentially lose their healing quality for the psyche. In contrast, for Jung, psychic conflict can be treated as something which is in service to the individuation process, and the symbols may be used not only to indicate something about the psychic conflict in order to resolve it but also, through their teleology, say something about how relating to the opposites symbolically can lead to greater wholeness.

Langs tends to treat symbols as puzzles to be solved, not as positive products of the psyche which allow psychic life to articulate its own form—indeed, its own psychological and adaptive environment—whereas Jung thinks that it is the symbolizing function which brings meaning to life. Though in the first phase of analysis ("reductive" phase), trigger decoding symbols would be necessary, for Jung this reduction is done ultimately so that the symbolic material can be rearticulated in a new set of symbols, a set more apt to the process of individuation and the later ("synthetic") phase of analysis (Jung, 1948). Similarly, though it is possible Jung would accept at least some of Langs' strictures on the analytic frame, in the end, the frame itself must also become part of the psychological reality of the analytic relationship, a living part of the analytic third. In essence, the value of Langs' work from Jung's point of view would probably not refer to analysis as an entire process, but only to the earlier phases of the process.

This suggests that, from a technical point of view, some of the basic principles Langs articulates are not to be taken as comprehensive principles of analysis, but as applicable primarily to the beginning and reductive phase of analytic work. However, this further suggests that if, like Jung, we understand analysis to be not only about a reductive phase but also about the synthetic phase of aiding the patient toward a fuller symbolic life and a living wholeness, Langs' method will have much less relevance later in the process.[9]

Individual and Collective

A further area where Jung's theories potentially illuminate the clinical problem of adaptation is with regard to what he terms the "collective unconscious." It would take us too far afield to tackle either the entire problem of the meaning of "collective" in Jung—something which probably merits a book-length study of its own[10]—or all the ways in which issues associated

9. Goodheart also notes that Langs has not "explored deeply the nature of therapy once the secured-symbolizing field is firm" (1980: p. 34). That comment would appear to be equally true of Langs' later work.

10. In a nutshell, "collective" in Jung can refer to basically anything not individual—which is clearly too large a categorization to be a theoretically useful concept. For example, "collective" can, among other things, refer to (1) something being general in the sense of being an essential feature of human nature; (2) historically contingent but widespread social phenomena, like Nazism or capitalism (which is clearly not "collective" in the first sense); or (3) archetypal realities, which appear to be universal in something like the first sense but yet transpersonal, extra-empirical, and divine or divine-like. Furthermore, each of these meanings have different opposites, if one thinks them through, demonstrating just how different each of these mean-

with collectives impact adaptation. Nonetheless, the role of collectives in adaptive problems is too important to be sidestepped entirely.

Jung envisions individual psychic life as something comprised of both individual and collective dimensions. In practice, this means that the psychic life of a human individual must be understood both in terms of individual psychology and also as in part a product of the collective social units of which the person is a part, both as subjective experience and as psychic environment in which and toward which the individual is adapting. Further, according to Jung, the social units of which an individual is a part each possess what we might term a "group mind" or "psychic ethos," one which typically, substantially, and to some extent unconsciously impacts an individual's psychic life and experience. Hence the psyche is not only a locus of individual experiences but also a sensorium for collective experiences, values, and so forth.

This theoretical stance on Jung's part helps us to understand why he seems at times to equivocate on terms of great importance in his theories. For example, we have seen that Jung has two, mostly incompatible meanings of "adaptation": a positive sense referring to a basic dynamism in the psyche at the service of individuation and a second, negative sense referring to the extent to which a person is too collectively minded, something which he views as typically inimical to individuation. We have similarly seen that Jung seems to have two meanings of "individuation": one meaning "becoming whole," the other meaning "differentiated from the collective." While each of these might be positive goals, the meaning of the terms is clearly different and not entirely coextensive. Yet we can begin to see at this point some of the reasons why Jung falls prey to these theoretical equivocations.

Jung understandably tends to use the second meaning of "individuation" ("differentiated from the collective") when he is focusing on the external, social aspects of individuation. After all, individuation, though a goal of human life, is not necessarily pursued by everyone and therefore the individual pursuing it will tend to "stick out in a crowd," because such a person will tend to live in a way which contrasts with at least some collective values. In contrast, Jung tends to use the first meaning of "individuation" ("becoming whole") when he is viewing it exclusively from a standpoint internal to the individual psyche (i.e., in abstraction from the social context). Similarly, when Jung uses "adaptation" in a positive (dynamic) sense of the term, it emphasizes the first and primary meaning of individuation, since it refers to the kind of adaptation that functions in the service of being whole and undivided and, further, because this meaning describes the psyche from an internal standpoint. When Jung uses "adaptation" in the negative sense of being too "collectively minded,"

---

ings is from the others. Thus, the term "collective" should, in most cases, only be used with appropriate qualifications, such as delineating in which sense it is being used. Here it is being used in the second sense.

it is understood to be the opposite of the second sense of individuation, being differentiated from the collective, and is also being used in the social as opposed to the internal sense. The fact that both terms, individuation and adaptation, are at times used from an internal standpoint and, at other times, from a social standpoint explains why Dieckmann and others have misread Jung on adaptation and individuation: they didn't recognize which specific sense of individuation was being used in reference to, and at times in contrast to, which sense of adaptation.

Yet if we move beyond the purely conceptual issues and try to understand why Jung conflated these different meanings of individuation and adaptation, it appears to be because of the paradoxical fact that the psyche is *ontologically* individual, yet *experientially* both individual and collective. In other words, though the psyche must be conceived as an individual and real being ("reality of the psyche"), it *experiences* itself not only as an individual but also as a sensorium of collective experiences. Consequently, the individual person seeking wholeness must not only be in contact with their own unconscious processes but must also sift through individual relationships as well as memberships within their various significant communities and collectives, in order to make such relationships conscious and recognize the *social* shadow residing in one's unconscious, alongside the individual shadow. When individuation and adaptation are viewed exclusively from the standpoint internal to the psyche, the issues associated with the collective unconscious tend to fall through the cracks, whereas when individuation and adaptation are viewed in the second, social senses of the terms, they tend to highlight the collective factor.

It would be difficult for Langs to treat this specific issue, in part because he has no equivalent to the "collective" in his understanding of the psyche and in part because he would tend to think that, in any case, he is only concerned with the individual's adaptive problems, whether bound up with social issues or not. While that all might be true, it would leave out the fact that Langs would be understanding the "collective" as in some sense external to the individual psyche—at least if it poses an adaptive problem. Jung, in contrast, sees individual psychic experience *itself* as at least at times co-constituted by social mores and collective, psychic ethoses; hence, the "adaptive context" is not exactly an outer or an inner one but is in some sense and to some extent both. Consequently, Jung requires a different approach to the collective dimension of psychic life, his "archetypal approach," according to which more general factors of a collective psyche are delineated and understood through collective symbols.

One way of understanding this set of problems clinically is in terms of Hartmann's image of "equilibrium." Though, as we saw in chapter 2, Hartmann delineates four different kinds of equilibrium in terms of which he wants to understand healthy adaptation, we also note that Hartmann does not explicitly refer to the *human* environment as the chief locus of adaptive issues. For our purposes, therefore, we can emphasize, either as a fifth form of psychic equilibrium or as a specification to the first form Hartmann outlines, an equilibrium between the psyche and the social, collective environment.

Understood in this way, we could say that the "psyche-social environment equilibrium" consists in balancing the aims and values of individual pursuits with the aims and values of the specific community or collective, always guided by one's impulse toward, and understanding of, one's individuation process. This balancing is itself in principle adaptive and subject to new adaptive contexts when new factors emerge within a determinate range of possibilities. The specific application of this principle is highly personal, bound up with how the value hierarchies of each side of the tension seem to merge into a relatively coherent unity. Nonetheless, this balancing appears to be a genuine principle of psychic life and thus to have clinical relevance, at least insofar as we admit that to be a flourishing and individuated human being also requires that one learn how to live cooperatively and in community with others, without being unconsciously swept into the collective ethos. Indeed, it is right here where we meet the tension mentioned in chapter 2, namely, that we at times need to recognize a higher standard of value than that of adaptation, especially when collective values are either a hindrance or, worse, inimical to the individuation process of a person.

While we cannot enter into the vast set of clinical problems these points suggest, it is still important to note them because they are quite central for how we work with the adaptive issues of our patients. It makes quite a difference if we are dealing with a patient who, for example, is suffering from the consequences of some false idealizations versus the case of someone with the same issues but whose false idealizations tend to be derived from and confirmed by significant social collectives—whether familial, professional, national, or what have you—and thus is battling not only with individual issues but with relevant and influential collectives whose collective psychic power seem to confirm those idealizations. An overvaluation of the collective, for example, or the opposite, an overvaluation of one's own experience in contrast to the collective, can each be a clinical issue.

Concretely, these issues of individual versus collective adaptation particularly emerge where powerful collective factors are also deeply pathological and impinge strongly on individual patients, amplifying adaptive problems in significant ways. For example, the advertising industry in part lives off robust images of happiness based on material possessions, something which greatly impacts the average American therapy patient. The implicit and exaggerated promises of happiness wrought by consumer capitalism produce in our patients existential questions about what happiness really means and whether happiness is attainable, and it also colonizes the psyche of many of our patients with a profound resentment, based on the promises of happiness from consumption which experience only rarely confirms. This is just an example and surely not the only social pathology to watch for clinically. Yet it illustrates a general problem for our understanding of adaptation, namely: what counts as healthy, "normal" adaptation?[11] Indeed, how healthy and normal can adaptation be if the collectives to which one is adapting are pathological?[12]

It is most likely for this latter reason that Jung understood individuation to be not only about wholeness but also about differentiating from social collectives. In this respect, Jung was very much a part of a European intellectual milieu of his time, in which social theorists, philosophers, theologians, and others were criticizing the rise of so-called mass society and were concerned that genuine individuality was being subsumed into unconscious collectivity. The problems they saw in a glass darkly are, if anything, intensified in our time, a century later.

It is a clinically important task to recognize where adaptive material may be expressing not only individual issues and pathologies but also collective issues and/or pathologies. It can further be stated as a clinical principle that healthy adaptation requires a sense for social pathologies which, if possible, we should aid the patient in bringing to consciousness, in the hopes that the patient will gain the insight that such pathologies should be avoided where possible. When it is not possible to avoid them entirely, aiding a patient to make a clear, conscious decision of the extent to which they are willing to conform psychic life and behavior to recognized social pathology and for what reason is called for. Not to do so runs a number of potential risks for the patient, the extreme case being producing a figure like Eichmann: the kind of person who adapts himself so well to social pathology that he is "just doing his job," while he destroys the lives of thousands of people.

Adaptation, Clinical Interaction, and Ethics

In chapter 1, we expressed appreciation of Langs' and Jung's advancements in the development and understanding of clinical interaction within the depth psychological tradition but also the conviction that Max Scheler does a better job of articulating philosophically what occurs in the interactive field than either Langs or Jung. There are many implications of Scheler's conception of psychic interaction whose development would go far beyond the aims of this study, ranging over questions of how to differentiate the often too vague conceptions of "mental" life in analytic literature, to issues of what role spirit and lived body should play in analytic process, to the parallel's in Scheler's conception to the literature on the "analytic third," and others. For our

---

11. This in principle raises important questions for quantitative research, especially when the "statistical mean" is treated as "normal." If the social collective is deeply pathological as a whole, what counts as the statistical mean will tend to be so as well—one of the serious ethical problems around attempts at "value-free" research in the human sciences.

12. We have looked at some of the specific problems associated with the collective values of consumer capitalism in White (forthcoming a) and well as some associated with the recent pandemic in White (forthcoming b). For a broader discussion of working with individuals when the collective displays signs of pathology, see Tuley and White (forthcoming).

purposes, it is worth mentioning only a few points relevant to problems associated with adaptation.

First of all, Langs, as we have seen, emphasizes adaptation to external stimuli, a viewpoint which permitted him to see very clearly that analysis and therapy are processes of mutual adaptation between patient and clinician. For this reason, Langs emphasizes not only transference-countertransference phenomena in his adaptive theory, but also the extent to which there are potentially valid perceptions occurring in the clinical relationship. Hence there is always a fairly complicated process of differentiation going on in Langs' approach, as one attempts to discern both: (1) the duality of the patient's experience of both valid and invalid (transference) experiences and (2) the duality of the analyst's or therapist's experience of valid and invalid (countertransference) experiences. All four of these experiential directions have their places in the process, according to Langs' approach, and all have to be taken into account.[13]

This approach of Langs can be quite helpful in certain respects, especially as one attempts to sift through diverse material and to understand its various layers of meaning. Further, one of Langs' goals in delineating the complex interaction within the therapeutic dyad is to highlight areas in which a therapist may be defending against material potentially critical of the therapist, reducing it to a mere invalid transference on the part of the patient. Especially for the budding analyst-in-training, this can be a helpful way of elucidating different aspects of the material and highlighting the ruthless honesty an analyst needs to have with themselves.

At the same time, it behooves us to notice that language of this kind—"valid" versus "invalid" perception—is a quasi-scientific language, suggesting that there are either valid, true, genuine perceptions in the clinical interaction or invalid, false, deceptive perceptions: each is one or the other. The unconscious background to this sort of approach appears to be the true-false opposition, which suggests what in philosophy would be called a "contradictory relationship" (i.e., an either-or-with-nothing-in-between sort of relationship). Clinically speaking, this seems to be something of a far-fetched assumption, namely, that experiences on either the analyst's or the patient's part can be parsed into categorial distinctions of this kind, as if clinical experiences are simply one thing or another. Furthermore, we should not miss the familiar attitude out of which this approach appears to be arising. As discussed in a previous section, Langs tends to take symbols, which are multivalent, and transform them into straightforward, monovalent, and literal statements, as if such a translation of symbol is sufficient to understand its meaning. In a given moment, that indeed may be sufficient. But to understand a whole

---

13. In principle, Langs' approach includes an even more complicated (six-fold) schema than this, which he has articulated (1982). We have not attempted to analyze that schema, however, in part because it does not seem to have greatly impacted the rest of Langs' work, even though it was posed in arguably the *magnum opus* of the first half of his career.

clinical interaction in terms of this four-fold directionality strikes this author and clinician as too simplistic.

For one, since, as a rule, especially the unconscious material we are after in analytic sorts of therapy is expressed symbolically, why reduce multivalent material to merely two valences, valid and invalid? Further, there appears to be no good reason to think that either the supposedly valid or supposedly invalid is entirely one or the other, because there could be implications of each within any given piece of material. Sometimes, for example, imaging something in one way might exaggerate one point but underrate another; in what sense is that image valid or invalid? In the case of Bruce, a part of his unconscious image linked this clinician to the patient's abusing teacher and the supervisor to the psychologist; are those images expressing valid or invalid perceptions? Depending on the criteria used, it would appear to be both. Indeed, we might wonder by what criteria we make any such judgment. In any case, whatever counts as "valid" and "invalid" could be equally helpful and valuable for analytic work, depending on what one does with the material, raising the question of what exact utility there is in naming some perception valid versus invalid. Hence, though one important point Langs means to underline by this differentiation should not be lost on us— that those of us working from the chair of the analyst or therapist may be tempted to defend against implicit criticisms of ourselves and our work in patient material—it appears as a whole that there is a certain lack of subtlety in Langs' approach here.

Part of this lack of subtlety arises from Langs' insistence that adaptation is always about an outer adaptive context. Because of this presupposition, he can only read clinical material in terms of adaptations arising either from the patient adapting to the analyst or the analyst adapting to the patient. Yet, while Langs deserves credit for recognizing the importance of mutual adaptation in sessions and in therapeutic process, there appears to be a good deal more going on than his picture suggests. For one, as we pointed out, valid and invalid are inadequate descriptors for symbolic material. Furthermore, one could add to this point Jung's idea that there are really six distinct relationships which need to be accounted for in the clinical interaction: the relationships between conscious and unconscious in both analyst and patient; the relationship between the consciousness of each; the relationships between unconscious of each to the consciousness of the other; and the relationship between the unconscious dimension of each. Any attempt to define "valid" versus "invalid" in the midst of all that will likely fall either on the Scylla of oversimplification or the Charybdis of being too complicated to be of much use in the clinical setting.

More important for our purposes, however, is that the clinical interaction is not well-described in terms of just two parties, analyst or therapist and patient. In addition to the clinical dyad, what Ogden has termed the "analytic third" is always already present, a kind of psychic field and context, as described chapter 1, in which the interaction occurs. Though Jung's most insightful reading of this third is greatly complicated for your average analytic reader by being found in his interpretations of alchemical texts, it is not without reason that Jung approached the issue in this way. The complexity of this relationship is in many ways treated better in terms of images—precisely because of their multivalence—than in terms of straightforward propositions. Jung's treatment of the datum that has become known as the "analytic third" also suggests a further point: that the dyad not only constitutes a mutually produced psychic field from the start, but that the material in the third can be considerably different from the material in each party (Ogden, 2004; Cwik, 2006; Cwik, 2011). It is truly a third thing, not just the sum of the expressed content of the two psyches involved.

Another way to describe this situation is to say that the third constitutes a further adaptive context in therapy and analysis. Perhaps because of Langs' materialistic tendencies, he only considers materially based factors related to the clinical setting, such as fee, setting, privacy (in a physical room), etc., plus the other person in the room as the adaptive context in therapy. Yet Jung's final articulation of the transference in *Psychology of the Transference* as well as Ogden's and Cwik's work, respectively, all indicate that there is also a third which counts as both a new adaptive context and a psychic environment in which, to which, and according to which each of the members of the clinical dyad is also adapting, thus indicating a substantial adaptive context more or less wholly missing from Langs' analysis of the clinical situation.

This being the case, Lang's assumptions about clinical interaction are in certain respects inadequate for articulating the basic clinical factors he seeks to understand. Under no circumstances does it seem adequate to assume that there is only a mutual, external adaptation of each party to the other going on in the interaction. The third is neither of the two parties and its contents are more than the sum of its parts; nor is the analytic third either clearly external or internal to either the psyche of the analyst or that of the patient, such that Langs' model of exclusively external adaptive triggers does not obviously apply to it. As our discussions concerning the frame as well as our considerations concerning the third in chapter 1 indicate, much of the work in analysis early on in the process consists in differentiating the aspects of the entire clinical field, determining what aspects are the patient's, what aspect the analyst's, and what aspects consist of something mutually produced but different from each. Furthermore, any attempt to reduce these contents to valid and invalid is equally inadequate, first because it makes no sense to assume symbols and images are valid or invalid, as if they can be treated like true or false propositions; second, because no matter what the contents of the images and symbols, they are certainly telling us something important about either or both of the persons involved or about the third that they produce, all of which can in principle be useful for analysis (Gill, 1984). Both Ogden's and Cwik's work in this area highlight how the appearance of seemingly irrelevant images nonetheless illuminate aspects of the analytic work unexpectedly, showing again that the terms such as "valid" and "invalid" are neither helpful nor descriptive of the actual psychic content in question.

While there are many more implications which might be drawn from the constitution of the analytic third, for our purposes what is crucial is to recognize that adaptive processes, associated with a responsiveness to clinical material, are key and that we cannot reduce the sets of adaptive processes occurring in session simply to a mutually external process of analyst to patient and vice versa. Indeed, the material in the case of Bruce suggests that the third in our work included, for example, a vague experience of threat to Bruce, something which, in hindsight, I noticed at times but could not understand until the watershed session outlined earlier, where the incidents with his teacher and with the child psychologist were revealed. Whether this experience on Bruce's part was evoked directly by me, by the setting, or by other factors is something we might speculate on and, at the time, I confess I didn't consider the issues in terms of the analytic third. Yet not only could it be done but a careful consideration of the images might well suggest a third sort of derivative communication from the two Langs' highlights.

It is right here in the interaction that we can recognize an important piece of therapeutic ethics. The material in sessions can be bound up primarily with the analyst, the patient, or the third, but in all cases we clinicians need to recognize that that material is often demanding of us that we expand into areas with which we may not feel comfortable—the basic gradient of our own adaptive process *as clinicians*. Jung's idea that we get the patients we need expresses this point, as does Searles' idea that our patients are always trying to make us the therapist they need. Langs seems to have recognized the ethical point to some extent, by highlighting the implicit critique of our work that might be present in the patient's material, a point that should be acknowledged. But what counts as the "material" of the session appears much larger, once the analytic third is acknowledged, and that material seems much more multivalent than Langs' four-fold division suggests. Further, the ethical dimension of this material is not only the implicit criticism that the material may imply, but the further demand that we activate adaptively the elements of ourselves that require development, to become the analyst the patient needs but also the analyst who can manage the analytic third. The analytic third potentially opens up many dimensions of the adaptive process, well beyond what can be treated here.

Conclusion

As a final point, though we have spent a good deal of time looking critically at Langs' thought throughout this chapter, the nature of those criticisms is of a peculiar kind. As a whole, the logic of those criticisms amounts to criticizing limits that Langs himself puts on his own theory. For example, linking Langs' adaptive paradigm to an entirely new and potentially foreign theory of adaptation, like that of Jung, in one sense undermines the foundations of the theory as Langs' conceived of it. However, as many of the comments in this chapter have emphasized, the criticisms of Langs' lack of sense for the "reality of the psyche" or of his failure to recognize the analytic third have been highlighted less to criticize Langs' clinical method but to expand its practice into areas he would not have thought of or imagined.

That Langs himself would likely not have approved of these expansions is not to be doubted. Langs' clinical model was largely derived from a natural scientific model; he sought to have a purely evidentially based practice, focusing on discrete clinical moments as the exclusive empirical basis of psychoanalytic practice. In contrast to Langs' view, we have argued that his method can and should be expanded beyond the very concrete orientation of his investigations, to the empirically more complex but nonetheless observable structural features of the psyche, such as Jung develops, as well as to the third that emerges within the clinical interaction.

Hence, if the argument of this study is basically correct, Langs' clinical method, at least the elements of it we have highlighted, is far more powerful and wide-ranging than he himself thought and the bulk of apparent limits to the method can be remedied through admitting from the outset the various factors associated with what Jung called "the reality of the psyche."

Bibliography

Adler, G. (n.d.). *Studies in analytical psychology*. New York: G. P. Putnam's Sons.

Baranger, M., and Baranger, W. (1966). Insight in the analytic situation. In R. Litman (ed.), *Psychoananlysis in the Americas* (pp. 56–72). New York: International Universities Press.

Beebe, J. (2017). *Energies and patterns in psychological type: The reservoir of consciousness*. London: Routledge.

Bion, W. (1970). *Attention and interpretation*. Windermere, FL: Tavistock.

Brooke, R. (2015). *Jung and phenomenology*. London: Routledge.

Burston, D. (2007). *Erik Erikson and the American. psyche. Ego, ethics and evolution*. Lanham, MD: Jason Aronson.

Cwik, A. (2006). Rosarium revisited. *Spring, 74*, 189–232.

Cwik, A. (2010). From frame through holding to container. In M. Stein (ed.), *Jungian psychoanalysis. Working in the spirit of C.G. Jung* (pp. 169–178). Chicago, IL: Open Court.

Cwik, A. (2011). Associative dreaming: Reverie and active imagination. *Journal of Analytical Psychology, 56*, 14–36.

Cwik, A. (2017). What is a Jungian analyst dreaming when myth comes to mind? Thirdness as an aspect of anima media natura. *Journal of Analytical Psychology, 62*(1), 107–29.

Dieckmann, H. (1991). *Methods in analytical psychology. An introduction*. Translated by B. Matthews. Asheville, NC: Chiron Publications.

Ellenberger, H. F. (2006). *The discovery of the unconscious: The history and evolution of dynamic psychiatry*. New York: Basic Books.

Erikson, E. (1964). *Insight and responsibility*. New York: Norton.

Fordham, M. (Ed.) (1974). *Technique in Jungian analysis*. Portsmouth, NH: William Heinemann Medical Books.

Fordham, M. (1978). Discursive review of Robert Langs' *The Therapeutic Interaction*, 2 vols. *Journal of Analytical Psychology, 23*(2), 193–96.

Freud, S. (1959/1911). Formulations regarding the two principles of mental functioning. In J. Riviere (ed.), *Sigmund Freud, Collected papers* (volume 4, pp. 13–21). New York: Basic Books.

Freud, S. (1959/1924). The loss of reality in neurosis and psychosis. In J. Riviere (ed.), *Sigmund Freud, Collected papers* (volume 2, pp. 277–82). New York: Basic Books.

Freud, S. (1962). *Three essays on the theory of sexuality*. Translated by J. Strachey. New York: Basic Books.

Gill, M. (1984). Robert Langs on technique: A critique. In J. Raney (ed.), *Listening and interpreting. The challenge of the work of Robert Langs* (pp. 395–413). Lanham, MD: Jason Aronson.

Goodheart, W. (1980). Theory of analytic interaction. *San Francisco Library Jung Institute Journal, 1*, 2–39.

Greenson, R. R. (1967). *The technique and practice of psychoanalysis*. New York: International Universities Press.

Grotstein, J. (1984). The higher implications of Langs's contributions. In J. Raney (ed.), *Listening and interpreting. The challenge of the work of Robert Langs* (pp. 3–20). Lanham, MD: Jason Aronson.

Hartmann, H. (1958). *Ego psychology and the problem of adaptation*. Translated by D. Rapaport. New York: International Universities Press.

Hodges, A. G. (1984). A Langsian approach to acting out. In J. O. Raney (ed.), *Listening and interpreting: The challenge of the work of Robert Langs* (pp. 75–97). Lanham, MD: Jason Aronson.

Hölscher, L. (2016). *The reality of the mind: Augustine's philosophical arguments for the human soul as a spiritual substance*. London: Routledge.

Jarrett, J. (1988). Jung's theory of functions: Some questions. In R. Papadopoulos (ed.), *Carl Gustav Jung: Critical assessments* (pp. 10–26). London: Routledge.

Jung, C. G. (1923). *Psychological types* (volume CW 6). Translated by R. F. C. Hull. Princeton, NJ: Princeton University Press.

Jung, C. G. (1923a). Psychological types. In *Psychological types* (volume CW 6, pp. 510–23). Translated by R. F. C. Hull. Princeton, NJ: Princeton University Press.

Jung, C. G. (1934). Basic postulates of analytical psychology. In *The structure and dynamics of the psyche* (volume CW 8, pp. 338–57). Translated by R. F. C. Hull. Princeton, NJ: Princeton University Press.

Jung, C. G. (1935). Principles of practical psychotherapy. In *The practice of psychotherapy* (volume CW 16, pp. 3–20). Translated by R. F. C. Hull. Princeton, NJ: Princeton University Press.

Jung, C. G. (1946). Psychology of the transference. In *The practice of psychotherapy* (volume CW 16, pp. 163–323). Translated by R. F. C. Hull. Princeton, NJ: Princeton University Press.

Jung, C. G. (1948). On psychic energy. In *The structure and dynamics of the psyche* (volume CW 8, pp. 3–65). Translated by R. F. C. Hull. Princeton, NJ: Princeton University Press.

Jung, C. G. (1952). *Symbols of transformation* (volume CW 5). Translated by R. F. C. Hull. Princeton, NJ: Princeton University Press.

Jung, C. G. (1953). *Two essays on analytical psychology* (volume CW 7). Translated by R. F. C. Hull. Princeton, NJ: Princeton University Press.

Jung, C. G. (1955). The philosophical tree. In *Alchemical studies* (volume CW 13, pp. 251–349). Translated by R. F. C. Hull. Princeton, NJ: Princeton University Press.

Jung, C. G. (1955a). The theory of psychoanalysis. In *Freud and psychoanalysis* (volume CW 4, pp. 83–226). Translated by R. F. C. Hull. Princeton, NJ: Princeton University Press.

Jung, C. G. (1959). *Aion: Researches into the phenomenology of the self* (volume CW 9ii). Translated by R. F. C. Hull. Princeton, NJ: Princeton University Press.

Jung, C. G. (1968). *Analytical psychology: Its theory and practice. The Tavistock lectures*. London: Routledge & Kegan Paul.

Jung, C. G. (1977). Adaptation, individuation, collectivity. In *The symbolic life* (volume CW 18, pp. 449–54). Princeton, NJ: Princeton University Press.

Jung, C. G. (1989). *Memories, dreams, reflections*. New York: Vintage Books.

Kant, I. (1996). *Critique of pure reason*. Translated by W. S. Pluhar. Indianapolis, IN: Hackett.

Kugler, P. H., J. (1985). The autonomous psyche. A communication to Goodheart from the bi-personal field of Paul Kugler and James Hillman. *Spring*, 141–63.

Langs, R. (1976). *The bipersonal field*. Lanham, MD: Jason Aronson.

Langs, R. (1978). *The listening process.* Lanham, MD: Jason Aronson.

Langs, R. (1978a). *Technique in transition.* Lanham, MD: Jason Aronson.

Langs, R. (1979). *The therapeutic environment.* Lanham, MD: Jason Aronson.

Langs, R. (1980). *Interactions: The realm of transference and countertransference.* Lanham, MD: Jason Aronson.

Langs, R. (1982). *Psychotherapy: A basic text.* Lanham, MD: Jason Aronson.

Langs, R. (1992). 1923: The advance that retreated from the architecture of the mind. *International Journal of Communicative Psychoanalysis & Psychotherapy, 7*(1), 3–15.

Langs, R. (2004). *Fundamentals of adaptive psychotherapy and counseling.* London: Macmillan Palgrave.

Langs, R. (2004a). Death anxiety and the emotion-processing mind. *Psychoanalytic Psychology, 21*(1), 31–53.

Langs, R. (2005). The challenge of the strong adaptive approach. *Psychoanalytic Psychology, 22*(1), 49–68.

Langs, R. (2010). *Freud on a precipice: How Freud's fate pushed psychoanalysis over the edge.* Lanham, MD: Jason Aronson.

Langs, R., and Searles, H. (1980). *Intrapsychic and interpersonal dimensions of treatment: A clinical dialogue.* Lanham, MD: Jason Aronson.

Lothane, Z. (1997). Freud and the interpersonal. *International Forum of Psychoanalysis, 6,* 175–84.

Lothane, Z. (2003). What did Freud say about persons and relations? *Psychoanalytic Psychology, 20,* 609–17.

Lothane, Z. (2009). Dramatology in life, disorder, and psychoanalytic therapy: A further contribution to interpersonal analysis. *International Forum of Psychoanalysis, 18*(3), 135–48.

Lothane, Z. (2010). The analysand and analyst practicing reciprocal free association—defenders and deniers. *International Forum of Psychoanalysis, 19,* 155–64.

Lothane, Z. (2011). Dramatology vs. narratology: A new synthesis for psychiatry, psychoanalysis, and interpersonal drama therapy (IDT). *Archives of Psychiatry and Psychotherapy, 4,* 29–43.

Merleau-Ponty, M. (2002). *Phenomenology of perception.* London: Routledge.

Mills, J. (2012). *Conundrums: A critique of contemporary psychoanalysis.* London: Routledge.

Mills, J. (2014). *Underworlds.* Milton Park: Taylor & Francis.

Milner, M. (1952). Aspects of symbolism in comprehension of the not-self. *International Journal of Psycho-analysis, 33,* 181–95.

Mitchell, S. (1988). *Relational concepts in psychoanalysis: An integration.* Cambridge, MA: Harvard University Press.

Ogden, T. (1997). Reverie and metaphor: Some thoughts on how I work as a psychoanalyst. *The International Journal of Psycho-analysis, 78,* 719–32.

Ogden, T. (2004). The analytic third. Implications for psychoanalytic theory and technique. *The Psychoanalytic Quarterly, 73*(1), 167–94.

Quenk, A. Q., N. (1982). The use of psychological typology in analysis. In M. Stein (ed.), *Jungian Analysis.* Chicago, IL: Open Court.

Raney, J. (Ed.). (1984). *Listening and interpreting: The challenge of the work of Robert Langs.* Lanham, MD: Jason Aronson.

Rapaport, D. G., and Gill, M. M. (1959). The points of view and assumptions of metapsychology. *International Journal of Psycho-analysis, 40,* 153–62.

Scheler, M. (1973). *Formalism in ethics and non-formal ethics of values*. Translated by M. Frings. Evanston, IL: Northwestern University Press.

Scheler, M. (1973a). Ordo Amoris. In *Selected Philosophical Essays* (pp. 98–135). Translated by D. Lachterman. Evanston, IL: Northwestern University Press.

Scheler, M. (1981). *Man's place in nature*. Translated by H. Meyerhoff. New York: Farrar, Straus and Giroux.

Scheler, M. (2017). *The nature of sympathy*. London: Routledge.

Seifert, J. (1973). *Leib und seele: Ein beitrag zur philosophischen anthropologie*. Salzburg, Austria: Anton Pustet.

Sharp, D. (1987). *Personality types: Jung's model of typology*. Ontario: Inner City Books.

Stavish, M. (2018). *Egregores: The occult entities that watch over human destiny*. Rochester, VT: Inner Traditions.

Stein, M. (1998). *Transformation: The emergence of the self*. College Station, TX: Texas A & M University Press.

Tuley, L. C. W. J. (Ed.). (Forthcoming). *When the world is on fire. Jungian analysis at the nexus of individual and collective trauma*. London: Routledge.

Wampold, B. (2001). *The great psychotherapy debate: Models, methods, and findings*. Mahwah, NJ: Lawrence Erlbaum Associates.

Wampold, B. (2010). *The basics of psychotherapy: An introduction to theory and practice*. Washington, DC: American Psychological Association.

White, J. (2001). Max Scheler's tripartite anthropology. *Proceedings of the American Catholic Philosophical Association*, 255–66.

White, J. (2005). Exemplary persons and ethics. The place of St. Francis in the philosophy of Max Scheler. *American Catholic Philosophical Quarterly*, 79(1), 57–90.

White, J. (2007). Lived body and ecological value cognition. In S. H. Cataldi and W. S. Hamrick (eds.), *Merleau-Ponty and environmental philosophy: Dwelling on the landscapes of thought* (pp. 177–89). Albany, NY: SUNY Press.

White, J. (2008). Divine light and human wisdom: Transcendental elements in Bonaventure's illumination theory. *International Philosophical Quarterly*, 48(2), 175–85.

White, J. (2009). Illuminating Josef Seifert's theory of a priori knowledge in back to things in themselves. On what—and how—we learn from St. Bonaventure's illumination theory. In *To love all truth and in all things* (pp. 113–56). Santiago, Chile: Ediciones UC.

White, J. (2011). St. Bonaventure and the problem of doctrinal development. *American Catholic Philosophical Quarterly*, 85(1), 177–202.

White, J. (2012). Person and environment. Vital sympathy and the roots of environmental ethics. In J. M. W. Sanders (ed.), *Ethics and phenomenology* (pp. 221–40). Lanham, MD: Lexington Books.

White, J. (2013). Review of conundrums: A critique of contemporary psychoanalysis. *Journal of Analytical Psychology*, 58(4), 554–56.

White, J. (2014). Toward a phenomenology of participation mystique and a reformulation of Jungian philosophical anthropology. In M. Winborn (ed.), *Shared realities: Participation mystique and beyond* (pp. 220–44). Sheridan, WY: Fisher King Press.

White, J. (Forthcoming a). Colonizing the American psyche. Virtue and the problem of consumer capitalism. In L. C. W. J. Tuley (ed.), *When the world is on fire. Jungian analysis at the nexus of individual and collective trauma*. London: Routledge.

White, J. (Forthcoming b). The Jungian analyst in between life and death. Clinical ethics in an age of pandemic. In L. C. W. J. Tuley (ed.), *When the world is on fire. Jungian analysis at the nexus of individual and collective trauma*. London: Routledge.

White, J. (Forthcoming c). On the psyche of psychoanalysis. Scheler's contribution to psychoanalytic clinical theory and practice. In L. C. W. J. Tuley (ed.), *When the world is on fire. Jungian analysis at the nexus of individual and collective trauma*. London: Routledge.

Winborn, M. (2019). *Interpretation in Jungian analysis. Art and technique*. London: Routledge.

Index

aberration, 42–43

adaptation: "adaptive paradigm" of, 56; analytic listening and, 64–67, 81, 131; analytic relationship and, 59–61; analytic theory and, 4–6; being "too adapted" in, 85; biological, 47–48; clarifying Jung's, 106–8; clinical illustration of, 71–78; clinical interaction and, 38, 60–61, 71–77, 98–106, 123–24, 141–45; in clinical practice, 53–81, 98–106; clinical technique and, 109–46; communication and, 67–71, 130–32; communicative fields and, 62–64, 65, 71–76, 77, 132–33; compensatory function in, 85–86; conflict and, 46–47, 98–100, 136–37; defining, 9–10, 84–86; derivative communication and, 67–69, 76–78, 105–6; as descriptive, 84–85; as dynamic, 86; in early analytic theory, 39–51; in ego psychology, 44–49, 53–54; emotion and, 57, 57n2, 70; environment relating to, 43, 45–46, 139–41; Erikson and, 6–7, 7n2; ethics and, 141–45; as evaluative, 84–85; flexibility and, 37; Freud and, 40–44; goal of, 47–48; Hartmann and, 5, 44–51; human development and, 45–48, 86, 86n4; importance of, 1, 5–6, 55–56; individuation and, 6–7, 15, 38, 49, 86, 106–7, 130–31; introduction to, 9–11, 53–54; Jung and, 5, 6–7, 15, 15n3, 38, 39, 49–50, 60, 83–108, 96n11, 117–32; Langs and, 4–5, 53–81, 95–100, 107–8, 117–32, 145–46; through Langs' career, 53–59; Langs central ideas on, 59–71; life experiences and, 36–37; meanings and concepts of, 84–86; metapsychology and, 44–45, 50–51; original development of, 55–59; philosophy and, 10, 15; pleasure and, 40–42, 48; psyche and, 6–7, 9–38, 40–41, 43, 48–49, 84–86, 107, 117–40, 144, 146; in *On Psychic Energy*, 86–98, 107, 123; psychic life and, 3–4, 40–41, 124, 141–42; psychoanalytic theory and, 11, 22–35; psychodynamics and, 57–58; psychological equilibrium and, 46–49; psychological health and, 5, 9–10; psychological types and, 39; in *Psychology of the Transference*, 98–100, 136; reality and, 56–58; rigidity and, 37; sexuality and, 42–43; state of versus process of, 45, 47, 86–87; in therapeutic frame, 61, 61n6, 65, 133–36; trauma and, 78–80; unconscious and, 37–38, 59, 69–71, 74–75, 84–86, 119–21, 127–28; unconscious communication and, 64–71, 124, 130–31; value of, 125–28. *See also specific topics*

adaptive context: attitudinal, 96–97, 100; case presentations and, 1–4; change and, 96–97, 99–100, 125–26; communication and, 66; external, 95–98; images and, 1–4, 99–100; internal, 95–98; Jung on, 95–98; Langs on, 3–4, 55–59, 95–98, 122; trigger decoding in, 66, 137; unconscious and, 95–96, 119–20

adaptive triggers, 126–28

Adler, Gerhard, 109–12

Aeschylus, 21

affect, 92–94, 92n9

alloplastic alteration, 43, 46

analytic listening, 64–67, 81, 131

analytic theory: adaptation and, 4–6; adaptation in early analytic theory, 39–51; clinical technique in, 6–7; Freud and, 40–44, 46–49; Hartmann and, 44–51; images and, 2–3; on life experiences, 3; psyche in early analytic theory, 11–38

analytic third, 33, 33n11, 35, 38, 143–45

ancient philosophy, 21

archetype, 2, 120–21

attitudinal adaptive context, 96–97, 100

Augustine (Saint), 12–13, 89

authority figures, 73–77

autoplastic alteration, 43, 46

awareness: consciousness and, 20–22, 34, 37–38; of psyche, 31

balance, 139–40

Barangers' paper, 59–60

"Basic Postulates of Analytical Psychology" (Jung), 11–15

beauty, 40

behaviorism, 12–13

Beyond the Pleasure Principle (Freud), 48

biological adaptation, 47–48

body, 28–29

bull image, 1–2

Burston, Daniel, 7n2

capitalism, 140–41, 141n12

Cartesian theory, 18–19, 57

case presentations, 1–4

change, 96–100, 125–26

character, 37

clinical dyad, 33–35

clinical interaction: adaptation and, 38, 60–61, 71–77, 98–106, 123–24, 141–45; analytic third in, 33, 33n11, 35, 38, 143–45; Barangers' paper on, 59–60; with "Bruce,"

153

About the Author

John R. White, PhD, LPC, is a Jungian psychoanalyst and mental health counselor in private practice in Pittsburgh, Pennsylvania. He received his doctorate in philosophy in 1993 from the International Academy of Philosophy, in the Principality of Liechtenstein, an institution accredited through the Austrian university system. He received his diploma as a Jungian Psychoanalyst from the Interregional Society of Jungian Analysts in 2017. He is currently coordinator of the C. G. Jung Institute Analyst Training Program of Pittsburgh and president-elect of the Board of the Pittsburgh Psychoanalytic Center. He has more than thirty-five published articles, book chapters, edited volumes, and book reviews in both philosophy and psychoanalysis.